GUIDELINES

—— FOR ——

PULMONARY REHABILITATION PROGRAMS

AMERICAN ASSOCIATION OF CARDIOVASCULAR AND PULMONARY REHABILITATION

Gerilynn Connors, BS, RCP, RRT
St. Helena Hospital, Napa Valley, CA

Lana Hilling, RCP
Mt. Diablo Medical Center, Concord, CA

Editors

Human Kinetics Publishers

Library of Congress Cataloging-in-Publication Data

American Association of Cardiovascular & Pulmonary Rehabilitation.
   Guidelines for pulmonary rehabilitation programs / American
Association of Cardiovascular and Pulmonary Rehabilitation.
     p.   cm.
   Includes bibliographical references and index.
   ISBN 0-87322-402-7
   1. Lungs--Diseases, Obstructive--Patients--Rehabilitation-
-Standards. 2. Lungs--Diseases--Patients--Rehabilitation-
-Standards. 3. Respiratory therapy--Standards. I. Title.
   [DNLM: 1. Lung Diseases, Obstructive--rehabilitation.
2. Rehabilitation--standards. WF 600 A5117g]
RC776.03A64 1993
362.1'9624--dc20
DNLM/DLC
for Library of Congress   92-1572

ISBN: 0-87322-402-7

Photo Credits: Pages 1, 5, 8, 18, 20 (both), 30 (top), 52, 64 (top), 65 (both), and 68 by Trevor J. Murtagh; pages 4, 6 (both), 11, 12, 14 (top), 17, 25, 26, 30 (bottom), 31, 32, 33 (both), 37, 41, 42 (bottom), 44, 45 (bottom), 46, 49, 50 (bottom), 51, 55, 57, 63, 64 (bottom), 67, and 69 by Karen O'Brien; pages 14 (bottom), 19, 38, and 50 (top) by Steve Nobis; and pages 21, 22, 40 (both), and 42 (top) by Mark Herlinger.

Developmental Editor: Christine Drews; Assistant Editors: Laura Bofinger, Moyra Knight, Julie Swadener, and Dawn Roselund; Copyeditor: Wendy Nelson; Proofreader: Kathy Bennett; Indexer: Sheila Ary; Production Director: Ernie Noa; Typesetter: Ruby Zimmerman; Text Design: Keith Blomberg; Text Layout: Kimberlie Henris and Tara Welsch; Cover Design: Jack Davis; Interior Art: Kathy Fuoss; Printer: United Graphics

Printed in the United States of America   10 9 8 7 6 5

Human Kinetics
Web site: http://www.humankinetics.com/

United States: Human Kinetics, P.O. Box 5076, Champaign, IL 61825-5076
1-800-747-4457

Canada: Human Kinetics, Box 24040, Windsor, ON N8Y 4Y9
1-800-465-7301 (in Canada only)

Europe: Human Kinetics, P.O. Box IW14, Leeds LS16 6TR, United Kingdom
(44) 1132 781708

Australia: Human Kinetics, 57A Price Avenue, Lower Mitcham, South Australia 5062
(08) 277 1555

New Zealand: Human Kinetics, P.O. Box 105-231, Auckland 1
(09) 523 3462

Contents

Foreword

Rehabilitation was defined in 1942 by the Council of Rehabilitation as "the restoration of the individual to the fullest medical, mental, emotional, social and vocational potential of which he or she is capable." This process has been applied to patients with neuromuscular and musculoskeletal disorders for decades. More recently, individuals with cardiovascular or pulmonary disease have been considered by many as candidates for rehabilitation.

Most of those with lung dysfunction who participate in pulmonary rehabilitation programs have chronic obstructive pulmonary disease (COPD) with a combination of emphysema and chronic bronchitis. Although age-adjusted prevalence rates for COPD among men have been stable since 1980, with what appears to be a downward trend recently, the prevalence in women has increased.[1] Between 1969 and 1989, there has been a 54% increase in the age-adjusted death rate for COPD in the United States, compared to a 49% decrease for coronary artery disease.[2] In 1989, COPD was estimated to be the direct cause of death for 79,000 people in the U.S.[2]

Morbidity related to COPD is considerable. In 1989 in the U.S., an estimated 16 million office visits were made to physicians for COPD, and COPD was the first-listed diagnosis for 229,000 hospitalizations for COPD (unpublished data from the National Heart, Lung, and Blood Institute). Although hospitalizations for COPD have been decreasing in the last few years, office visits have continued to increase.[1] In the U.S., COPD is second only to coronary heart disease in the number of patients receiving Social Security disability payments because of their disease process.

The cost for health care in the U.S. is enormous, with an estimated $740 billion spent in 1991. The economic cost for COPD is also significant. In 1988, the direct cost for COPD for physicians' services, hospital care, and medications was estimated at $5.8 billion, the cost associated with morbidity at $3.8 billion, and the cost of lost productivity due to mortality at $3.6 billion (unpublished data from the National Heart, Lung, and Blood Institute). These estimates do not take into account the additional costs of human suffering.

Pulmonary rehabilitation can reduce the cost of health care by decreasing the need for hospitalizations for individuals with COPD,[3] and it provides many direct benefits to patients and their families, helping them to cope more effectively with the disease process.[4] Pulmonary rehabilitation should be considered for every patient with COPD. The common practice of reserving rehabilitation for patients with end-stage disease and severe limitation of function must change so that more individuals benefit from these programs.

Guidelines for Pulmonary Rehabilitation Programs represents a significant step forward in helping set the standards to which facilities offering these programs should adhere. They will help ensure that individuals with pulmonary impairment receive the quality of care they deserve. The American Association of Cardiovascular and Pulmonary Rehabilitation and those who contributed many hours of effort in developing these guidelines are to be commended for this major contribution to health care professionals and their patients.

John E. Hodgkin, MD
Medical Director, Respiratory Care and
Pulmonary Rehabilitation
Medical Director, Center for Health Promotion
St. Helena Hospital
Clinical Professor of Medicine
University of California, Davis

References

1. Feinleib M, Rosenberg HM, Collins JG, Delozier JE, Pokras R, Chevarley FM. Trends in COPD morbidity and mortality in the United States. *Am Rev Respir Dis.* 1989;140:S9-S18.
2. *National Heart, Lung, and Blood Institute Fact Book: Fiscal Year 1990.* US Dept of Health and Human Services. Public Health Service. National Institutes of Health, Feb. 1991.
3. Radovich J, Hodgkin JE, Burton GG, Yee AR. Cost-effectiveness of pulmonary rehabilitation. In: Hodgkin JE, Connors GL, Bell W, eds. *Pulmonary Rehabilitation: Guidelines to Success.* 2nd ed. Philadelphia, PA: J.B. Lippincott; 1992.
4. Hodgkin JE. Benefits and the future of pulmonary rehabilitation. In: Hodgkin JE, Connors GL, Bell W, eds. *Pulmonary Rehabilitation: Guidelines to Success.* 2nd ed. Philadelphia, PA: J.B. Lippincott; 1992.

Acknowledgments

The initial development of these guidelines took place at a weekend meeting in Cincinnati, Ohio, in September 1988 with William Bell, Gerilynn Connors, and Lana Hilling. The philosophy of pulmonary rehabilitation was discussed, and the groundwork was established. The purpose of writing this document was to establish nationally recognized pulmonary rehabilitation guidelines for program development, enhancement, and reimbursement.

The following individuals formed the guidelines committee and were the major writers of the document:

Editors

Gerilynn Connors, BS, RCP, RRT, Cochair
St. Helena Hospital
Napa Valley, CA

Lana Hilling, RCP, Cochair
Mt. Diablo Medical Center
Concord, CA

Committee Members

C. William Bell, PhD, MBA
Colorado Lung Center
Denver, CO

Kathleen Morris, RN, MS, RRT
St. Helena Hospital
Napa Valley, CA

Howard M. Kravetz, MD
Northern Arizona Chest Center
Prescott, AZ

Andrew L. Ries, MD
University of California, San Diego
San Diego, CA

The entire 1989–1991 board of directors of the AACVPR reviewed this document. The following people also provided revisionary comments: Mardi Barcena, RCP, Good Samaritan Hospital, San Jose, CA; Mary Burns, RN, BS, Little Company of Mary Hospital, Torrance, CA; Dawn Sassi-Dambron, RN, BSN, UCSD, San Diego, CA; Birgitta K. Ellis, PT, UCSD, San Diego, CA; Richard D. Falls, BSN, MS, St. Joseph's Hospital, Phoenix, AZ; Denise L. Frick, BS, RRT, McAuley Health Center, Ann Arbor, MI; Micki McAndrew Harman, RN, MSN, RRT, CCRN, Saudi Aramco, Dhahran; Tom LaFontaine, PhD, Missouri Heart Institute, Columbia, MO; Trina Limberg, BS, RRT, UCSD, San Diego, CA; Susan McInturff, RRT, RCP, Glasrock Home Health Care, Benicia, CA; James Maguire, PhD, RCP, Pall Biomedical, Glencove, NY; Roseann Myers, RN, UCSD, San Diego, CA; Judy Hartman Ruekberg, RN, Alvarado Hospital Medical Center, San Diego, CA; Douglas R. Southard, PhD, MPH, Assistant Professor of Health and Psychology, Virginia Tech, Blacksburg, VA; William Wilkison, RRT, BA, East Shore Rehabilitation Center, Harrisburg, PA.

An outside panel of nationally known pulmonary rehabilitation experts also served as reviewers before the final editing:

Allen I. Goldberg, MD
The Childrens Memorial Hospital
Chicago, IL

Edward L. Goldzimer, MD
Tri City Medical Center
Oceanside, CA

John E. Hodgkin, MD
St. Helena Hospital
Napa Valley, CA

Neil R. MacIntyre, MD
Duke University Medical Center
Durham, NC

Barry J. Make, MD
National Jewish Center for Immunology and Respiratory
   Medicine
Denver, CO

William F. Miller, MD
University of Texas, Southwest Medical Center
Dallas, TX

Thomas L. Petty, MD
Presbyterian/St. Luke's Center for Health Services Education
Denver, CO

Paul Selecky, MD
Hoag Memorial Presbyterian Hospital
Newport Beach, CA

Brian L. Tiep, MD
Casa Colina Center for Rehabilitation
Pomona, CA

Photos are printed with the courtesy of the pulmonary rehabilitation programs at Mt. Diablo Medical Center, Concord, CA, St. Helena Hospital, Napa Valley, CA, and the Colorado Lung Center, Denver, CO.

An educational grant from Glaxo Inc. (Allen & Hanburys) provided assistance in finalizing the document.

We want to express our gratitude to Debbie Duckett, who assisted with the clerical challenges as this project developed, and to Linda Hall, who found time in her busy schedule to review our manuscript at the copyediting stage.

We also give a special thank-you to *Beverly Striplin* and *Marie VanBeveren*, graduates and two very dedicated volunteers of the Pulmonary Rehabilitation Program of the Mt. Diablo Medical Center, Concord, CA, for their assistance in typing the many drafts of this manuscript.

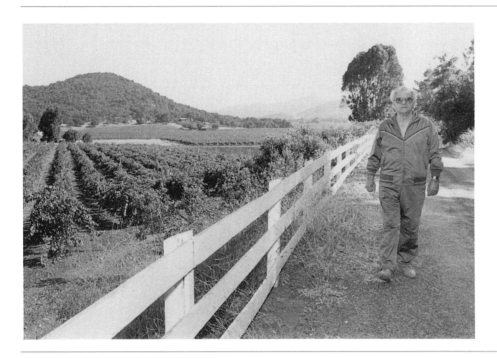

Chapter 1

Definition and Overview of Pulmonary Rehabilitation

Pulmonary rehabilitation has evolved over the past several decades in response to the dramatic increase in patients with chronic pulmonary diseases and the changing views of their medical needs. For many years, the standard of care for pulmonary patients included inactivity and rest. Patients were considered to be passive recipients of medical treatment. Pulmonary rehabilitation programs encourage the exact opposite to inactivity and rest. In most instances, inactivity and rest are counterproductive in optimizing lung health.

Many recent studies have demonstrated the benefits of pulmonary rehabilitation programs that involve patients actively in their own health care. Such programs have been developed based on sound preventive, therapeutic, and rehabilitative care principles with the goal of training patients in specific techniques and strategies to improve their functional capacity and to reduce the economic, medical, and social burdens of their diseases.[1-7]

Pulmonary rehabilitation was formally defined in 1974 by a committee of the American College of Chest Physicians.[8] Pulmonary physicians found a need to clarify the optimum type of care and treatment

> Pulmonary rehabilitation programs encourage activity and exercise to optimize lung health.

for pulmonary patients and to better define the role of rehabilitation. Since then, rehabilitation programs have grown to be an important component in the overall care of pulmonary patients. Health care providers have more options available for comprehensive care, and patients, families, and physicians do not have to be left alone to cope with the problems of chronic and often irreversible pulmonary diseases.

These guidelines are intended for a variety of readers:

- Professionals developing and updating pulmonary rehabilitation programs
- Physicians and other allied health care professionals referring patients for pulmonary rehabilitation
- Pulmonary rehabilitation providers working in existing programs
- Patients and significant others interested in a pulmonary rehabilitation program
- Third-party payors evaluating pulmonary rehabilitation programs
- Educators training health care professionals (nurses, physical therapists, respiratory therapists, physicians, etc.) about pulmonary rehabilitation

These guidelines, developed by the American Association of Cardiovascular and Pulmonary Rehabilitation (AACVPR), are intended to emphasize a number of issues related to pulmonary rehabilitation programs:

The AACVPR guidelines emphasize the individual needs of the patient.

- The rehabilitative care needs of the individual patient. These needs are determined collaboratively by the primary care physician, patient, and rehabilitation team (including the pulmonary rehabilitation medical director).
- Specific goals for each patient, delineated upon admission to the program.
- Regular evaluation of both patient performance and program components. Evaluation of patient progress is based on achievement of specific goals.
- A broad view, with regard to eligibility criteria, of indications and patient selection for program participation.
- The components of pulmonary rehabilitation, which include team assessment, patient training, exercise, psychosocial intervention, and follow-up.
- A focus on increasing the accessibility of pulmonary rehabilitation through earlier screening and detection of lung disease.
- Recommendations based on scientific studies, when available. References are cited to complement selected components of pulmonary rehabilitation.

Background Information

The evolution of pulmonary rehabilitation over the last quarter century reflects a changing view of health needs and health care for patients with chronic diseases. Beginning with the standard medical treatments included in pulmonary rehabilitation programs, professionals increasingly recognized the important interactions of psychological and emotional characteristics with physical attributes in determining a patient's overall health status.[1,9-12]

Pulmonary rehabilitation professionals recognize the importance of the interaction of psychological and emotional characteristics with physical attributes to determine optimal health.

Until well into the 1960s, the standard therapy for patients with chronic obstructive pulmonary disease (COPD: defined then as asthma, chronic bronchitis, and emphysema) was rest and avoidance of stress. One of the first studies to question this, by Pierce et al., demonstrated that reconditioning patients with COPD permits them to perform the same exercise levels with lower heart rate, respiratory rate, minute ventilation, and CO_2 production.[5,13] These physiological benefits occurred without change in pulmonary function and were found to be due, in part, to increased efficiency of motion and enhanced utilization of oxygen in exercising muscles.[13]

COPD has an insidious onset developing over a 20- to 30-year period with a long asymptomatic period. Early detection is important because early rehabilitation may prevent progression to chronic and disabling disease leading to increased morbidity and mortality associated with the later stages of lung disease (Appendix A. pp. 74-75).

The impact of chronic pulmonary diseases on morbidity and mortality has increased dramatically in recent decades in the United States and throughout the world. In the United States, COPD, which includes emphysema, chronic bronchitis, and allied conditions, ranks as the 5th leading cause of death as shown in Table 1.1 and the 2nd leading cause of long-term disability.[16-18] The number of people with COPD has increased 45.3% between 1979 and 1989. In contrast to the rates for heart and other major diseases, death rates from COPD have been increasing rapidly in the latter part of the 20th century. COPD has been estimated to affect approximately 10% to 20% of the adult population.[9,16,19-21]

> In the United States, COPD ranks as the 5th leading cause of death.

Table 1.1   Deaths From the Leading Causes, U.S., 1987

Total	2,123,000
1 Heart disease*	760,000
2 Cancer	477,000
3 Cerebrovascular disease (stroke)	150,000
4 Accidents	95,000
5 COPD and allied conditions	78,000
6 Pneumonia and influenza	69,000
7 Diabetes	39,000
8 Suicide	31,000
9 Chronic liver disease	26,000
10 Atherosclerosis	22,000
All other causes of death	376,000

*Includes 512,000 deaths from coronary heart disease.

Note. Reprinted with permission from ''Pulmonary Rehabilitation'' by G.L. Connors and J.E. Hodgkin. In *Respiratory Care: A Guide to Clinical Practice* (3rd ed.) (p. 656) by G.G. Burton, J.E. Hodgkin, and J.J. Ward (Eds.). Copyright 1991 by J.B. Lippincott.

Problems of morbidity from these diseases are even greater. The breathlessness, increasing cough, sputum production, and wheezing caused by chronic airflow limitation results in anxiety, apprehension, fear, as well as fatigue.[4] In reviewing the literature on the psychological characteristics of COPD patients, Dudley et al. pointed out that these patients tend to live in "emotional straightjackets," as all expressions of emotion lead to distressing or disabling symptoms.[4] Persons with respiratory disorders tend to be very nervous and tense, often fearful that their next breath will not come. Additionally, muscle tension stiffens the muscles of the chest wall, making breathing even more difficult. Consequently, COPD patients become deconditioned and unable to function independently.[22]

In addition to COPD,[23] asthma,[24] cystic fibrosis,[25] interstitial, occupational,[26] and environmental lung disease,[27] neuromuscular disease,[28] and pulmonary hypertensive and vascular diseases lead to progressive functional impairment and disability for increasing numbers of individuals. These diseases contribute significantly to morbidity and mortality, and pulmonary rehabilitation may be important for these patients as well. Other potential applications for pulmonary rehabilitation include rehabilitation of ventilator-dependent patients and the preparation and postoperative care of patients undergoing lung transplantation.[29]

Successful pulmonary rehabilitation requires that the patient and the multidisciplinary team members believe in the philosophy of pulmonary rehabilitation as outlined in the Code of Ethics on page 5. This philosophy should include a process that is directed toward the patient but occurs with the patient's cooperation. Pulmonary rehabilitation team members should serve as role models, in attitude, communication style, and professionalism, for the patient, significant others, and the general or medical community.

Pulmonary rehabilitation is an art of medical practice that attempts to return patients to their highest possible functional capacity.

Definition

In 1974, the American College of Chest Physicians' Committee on Pulmonary Rehabilitation adopted the following definition:[8]

> Pulmonary Rehabilitation may be defined as an art of medical practice wherein an individually tailored multidisciplinary program is formulated which through accurate diagnosis, therapy, emotional support, and education, stabilizes or reverses both the physio- and psychopathology of pulmonary diseases, and attempts to return the patient to the highest possible functional capacity allowed by his pulmonary handicap and overall life situation.

In 1981, the American Thoracic Society included this definition in its official position statement on pulmonary rehabilitation (see Appendix B).[30]

Outcomes

Pulmonary rehabilitation programs enhance standard medical care to control and alleviate symptoms and optimize functional capacity for patients with chronic pulmonary diseases. These programs have been studied most extensively for patients with COPD but have also been

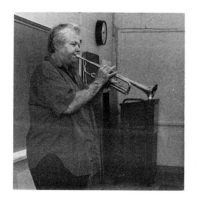

Code of Ethics for Pulmonary Rehabilitation Team Members

As pulmonary rehabilitation specialists involved in the care of people with lung impairment, we must strive, both individually and as a team, to maintain the highest ethical standards.

The principles set forth in this document outline the ethical and moral standards to which each pulmonary rehabilitation team member should conform.

The pulmonary rehabilitation specialist shall practice medically acceptable methods of pulmonary rehabilitation and shall not extend his/her practice beyond the competence and authority vested in him/her by the pulmonary rehabilitation medical director.

The pulmonary rehabilitation specialist shall always strive to increase and improve his/her knowledge and expertise and render to each pulmonary rehabilitation patient the full measure of his/her ability. All treatment modalities and training sessions shall be provided with respect for the dignity of the patient, unrestricted by considerations of social, economic, personal attributes, or religious beliefs.

The pulmonary rehabilitation specialist shall be responsible for the competent, efficient, and thorough performance of his/her designated duties.

The pulmonary rehabilitation specialist shall hold in strict confidence all privileged patient information.

The pulmonary rehabilitation specialist shall uphold the dignity and honor of the program through a strong belief and understanding of the objectives of pulmonary rehabilitation.

The pulmonary rehabilitation specialist, as a vital member of the health care team, shall strive for the prevention and early detection, not just the treatment, of pulmonary disease.

Note. Adapted from the American Association for Respiratory Care, Code of Ethics, 1986. 11030 Ables Lane, Dallas, TX 75229.

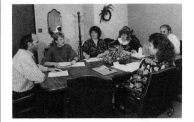

shown to be beneficial for patients with other types of pulmonary diseases.[23,29] There is substantial evidence that comprehensive pulmonary rehabilitation can produce demonstrated benefits.[30-35] Table 1.2 lists these beneficial outcomes.

Patient Goals and Program Goals

Pulmonary rehabilitation staff should be consistent in their understanding of the goals of pulmonary rehabilitation as it pertains to the individual patient and to the overall program. Pulmonary rehabilitation should be tailored to the needs of the individual patient once the initial assessment is complete. Patient-directed goals should be consistent

Table 1.2   Demonstrated Outcomes of Pulmonary Rehabilitation

Reduced hospitalizations and use of medical resources

Improved quality of life

Reduced respiratory symptoms (e.g., dyspnea)

Improved psychosocial symptoms (e.g., reversal of anxiety and depression and improved self-efficacy)

Increased exercise tolerance and performance

Enhanced ability to perform activities of daily living

Return to work for some patients

Increased knowledge about pulmonary disease and its management

Increased survival in some patients (i.e., use of continuous oxygen in patients with severe hypoxemia)

Note. Reprinted with permission from ''Position Paper of the American Association of Cardiovascular and Pulmonary Rehabilitation: Scientific Basis of Pulmonary Rehabilitation'' by A.L. Ries, 1990, *Journal of Cardiopulmonary Rehabilitation,* **10,** pp. 418-441. Published by J.B. Lippincott. Copyright 1990 by the American Association of Cardiovascular and Pulmonary Rehabilitation.

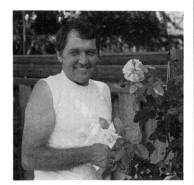

with the pulmonary rehabilitation definition and may include (but are not limited to) the following[30]:

- Control and alleviate, as much as possible, the symptoms and pathophysiological complications (pulmonary hypertension, etc.) of respiratory impairment.
- Train the patient to achieve her or his optimal capacity to carry out activities of daily living.
- Decrease psychological symptoms such as anxiety or depression.
- Improve quality of life.
- Return the patient to gainful employment when possible.
- Promote independence and self-reliance.
- Increase exercise tolerance.
- Reduce exacerbations and hospitalizations.
- Encourage participation in recreational pursuits.

The overall program goals may include the following:

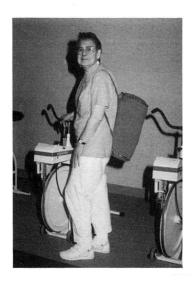

- Design and implement a patient's individualized program under the medical direction of a physician with special knowledge or interest in pulmonary rehabilitation.
- Train, motivate, and rehabilitate the patient to his or her maximum potential in self-care through an organized team effort.
- Train, motivate, and involve the patient's significant others in the patient's treatment program.
- Reduce the economic burden of pulmonary disease on society through reduction of acute exacerbations, hospitalizations, emergency room visits, long-term duration of convalescence, and possible return of the patient to gainful employment or active retirement.
- Educate the general public and health care professionals about pulmonary health and rehabilitation.
- Increase awareness in the medical community regarding the importance of early detection of pulmonary disease through screenings (e.g., spirometry).

- Increase awareness in the community about the harmful effects of smoking, secondhand smoke, and available treatment for effective smoking cessation.

Components

Essential components of comprehensive pulmonary rehabilitation are team assessment, patient training, exercise, psychosocial interventions, and follow-up. As shown in Figure 1.1, it is not simply an exercise or education program. Pulmonary rehabilitation team members must understand this concept in developing a complete and individualized program for the patient.

The essential components of pulmonary rehabilitation are team assessment, patient training, exercise, psychosocial intervention, and follow-up.

Figure 1.1
Essential Components of a Pulmonary Rehabilitation Program

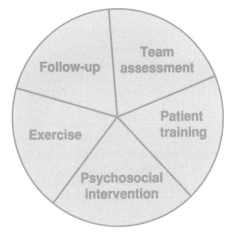

Team assessment*
PR medical director
Respiratory care practitioner
Nurse
Occupational therapist
Physical therapist
Exercise physiologist
Psychologist
Vocational counselor
Recreational therapist
Social worker
Nutritionist

Exercise
Exercise conditioning
Upper extremity strengthening
Respiratory muscle strengthening
Home program plan

Follow-up
Patient outcomes
Maintenance exercise group
Group meetings
Reevaluation as necessary

Patient training
Breathing retraining
Bronchial hygiene
Medications
Proper nutrition
ADL training
Panic control/relaxation
Energy conservation
Warning signs of infection
Sexuality for the pulmonary patient

Psychosocial intervention
Support system and dependency issues
Anger management
Treatment of depression
Counseling
Coping styles
Self-efficacy for rehabilitation-related behaviors
Impact of role change

*An individualized pulmonary rehabilitation program will meet the specific needs of the patient. Not every member of the pulmonary rehabilitation program team may be involved with the patient.

Note. Training or exercise alone does not constitute a pulmonary rehabilitation program. Reprinted with permission from "Organization and Management of a Pulmonary Rehabilitation Program" by L. Beytas and G.L. Connors. In *Pulmonary Rehabilitation: Guidelines to Success* (2nd ed.) by J.E. Hodgkin, G.L. Connors, and C.W. Bell (Eds.). Copyright 1992 by J.B. Lippincott.

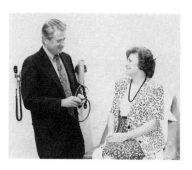

The essential components of pulmonary rehabilitation can be provided by the pulmonary rehabilitation team medical director and program director alone or in conjunction with a multidisciplinary team. The composition of the rehabilitation team will depend upon the facility and patient needs. Not every patient will need all of the multidisciplinary services mentioned in Figure 1.1, but these services should be available if needed.

The sequence for a comprehensive, individualized pulmonary rehabilitation program is depicted in Table 1.3. The following chapters expand on the sequence from initial patient selection to program follow-up.

Table 1.3 Sequence of Pulmonary Rehabilitation

1. Patient selection
2. Assess patient needs
3. Develop goals
4. Develop individualized treatment program
5. Assess the progress of goals achieved and the need for skilled level of care
6. Reassess the treatment program
7. Develop a home program plan for self-management and treatment
8. Determine patient follow-up needs and reassess for postprogram therapy

Note. Reprinted with permission from ''Organization and Management of a Pulmonary Rehabilitation Program'' by L. Beytas and G.L. Connors. In *Pulmonary Rehabilitation: Guidelines to Success* (2nd ed.) by J.E. Hodgkin, G.L. Connors, and C.W. Bell (Eds.). Copyright 1992 by J.B. Lippincott.

Conclusion

Pulmonary rehabilitation is a comprehensive treatment modality individualized to the patient's needs. The essential components of pulmonary rehabilitation include assessment, patient training, exercise, psychosocial intervention, and follow-up, and must be provided in a comprehensive program. Team understanding of the program goals and patient goals for pulmonary rehabilitation will allow optimum care for the respiratory patient, who has very specialized needs. In 1988, Dr. Hodgkin stated that an effective pulmonary rehabilitation program is no longer a luxury, but a necessity for lung patients.[36] This is even more true today.

The team's understanding of program goals and patient goals will result in optimum patient care.

References

1. Petty TL, Nett LM, Finigan MM, Brink GA, Corsello PR. A comprehensive care program for chronic airway obstruction: methods and preliminary evaluation of symptomatic and functional improvement. *Ann Intern Med*. 1969;70:1109-1120.
2. Mackey FG. Comprehensive rehabilitation care will take predominant place in delivery system. *Hospitals*. October 1, 1981;59-81.
3. Butts JR. Pulmonary rehabilitation through exercise and education. *CVP*. December/January 1981;17-21, 60-61.

4. Dudley DL, Glaser EM, Jorgenson B, et al. Psychosocial concomitants to rehabilitation in chronic obstructive pulmonary disease. *Chest*. 1980;77:413-544, 677.

5. Hughes RL, Davison R. Limitations of exercise reconditioning in cold. *Chest*. February 1983;2:241-249.

6. Berman LB, Sutton JR. Exercise for the pulmonary patient. *J Cardiopulmonary Rehab*. 1986;6:52-61.

7. Kaplan RM, Atkins CJ. Specific efficacy expectations mediate exercise compliance in patients with COPD. *Health Psychology*. 1984;3(3):223-242.

8. Petty TL. *Pulmonary Rehabilitation. Basics of RD*. New York, NY: American Thoracic Society; 1975.

9. Williams SJ. Chronic respiratory illness and disability: a critical review of the psychosocial literature. *Soc Sci Med*. 1989;28:791-803.

10. Cotes JE, Bishop JM, Capel LH, et al. Disabling chest disease: prevention and care: a report of the Royal College of Physicians by the College Committee on Thoracic Medicine. *JR Coll Physicians Lond*. 1989;15:69-87.

11. Lertzman MM, Cherniack RM. Rehabilitation of patients with chronic obstructive pulmonary disease. *Am Rev Respir Dis*. 1976;114:1145-1165.

12. Moser KM, Bokinsky GE, Savage RT, Archibald CJ, Hansen PR. Results of a comprehensive rehabilitation program: physiologic and functional effects on patients with chronic obstructive pulmonary disease. *Arch Intern Med*. 1980;140:1596-1601.

13. Pierce AK, Taylor HF, Archer RK, Miller WF. Responses to exercise training in patients with emphysema. *Arch Intern Med*. 1964;113:28-36.

14. Macklem PT, Permutt S. *The Lung in Transition Between Health and Disease*. New York, NY: Marcel Dekker, Inc; 1979.

15. Petty TL. The role for early identification of COPD. In: Hodgkin JE, Petty TL, eds. *Chronic Obstructive Pulmonary Disease: Current Concepts*. Philadelphia, PA: WB Saunders; 1987.

16. Higgins IT. Epidemiology of bronchitis and emphysema. In: Fishman AP, ed. *Pulmonary Diseases and Disorders*. 2nd ed. New York, NY: McGraw-Hill Book Co; 1988:1237-1246.

17. Higgins MW. Chronic airways disease in the United States: trends and determinants. *Chest*. 1989;96(suppl):328s-334s.

18. Lenfant C. Lung research: government and community. *Am Rev Respir Dis*. 1988;126:753-757.

19. Fletcher C, Peto R, Tinker C, Speizer FE. *The Natural History of Chronic Bronchitis and Emphysema*. Oxford, England: Oxford University Press; 1976.

20. Meuller RE, Kebe DL, Plummer J, Walker SH. The prevalence of chronic bronchitis, chronic airway obstruction, and respiratory symptoms in a Colorado city. *Am Rev Respir Dis*. 1971;103:209-228.

21. Woolcock AJ. Epidemiology of chronic airways disease. *Chest*. 1989;96(suppl):302-306.

22. Make B. COPD: management and rehabilitation. *Amer Family Phys*. 1991;43:1315-1324.

23. Foster S, Thomas HM. Pulmonary rehabilitation in lung disease other than COPD. *Am Rev Resp Dis*. 1990;141:601-604.

24. Hodgkin JE. United States audit of asthma therapy. *Chest*. 1986(suppl);90:625-665.

25. Orenstein DM. Cystic fibrosis. *Resp Care*. 1991;36(7):746-754.

26. Chan-Yeung M. Evaluation of impairment/disability in patients with occupational asthma. *Am Rev Resp Dis*. 1987;135:950-951.

27. Korn RJ, Dockery DW, Speizer FE, Ware JH, Ferris BG Jr. Occupational exposure and chronic respiratory symptoms: a population-based study. *Am Rev Respir Dis*. 1987;136:298-304.

28. Owen RR. Postpolio syndrome and cardiopulmonary conditioning. In: *Rehabilitative Medicine: Adding Life to Years* (special issue). *West J Med*. 1991;154:557-558.

29. Squires RW, Allison TG, Miller TD, Gan GT. Cardiopulmonary exercise testing after unilateral lung transplantation: a case report. *J Cardiopulmonary Rehabil*. 1991;11:192-196.

30. Hodgkin JE, Farrell MJ, Gibson SR, et al. Pulmonary rehabilitation: official ATS statement. *Am Rev Respir Dis*. 1981;124:663-666.

31. Hodgkin JE, Branscomb BV, Anholm JD, et al. Benefits, limitations and the future of pulmonary rehabilitation. In: Hodgkin JE, Zorn EG, Connors GL, eds. *Pulmonary Rehabilitation: Guidelines to Success*. Boston, Mass: Butterworth; 1984.

32. Burton GG, Gee G, Hodgkin JE, Dunham JL. Cost effectiveness studies in respiratory care: an overview and some possible early solutions. *Hospitals*. 1975;49:61-71.

33. Hudson LD, Tyler ML, Petty TL. Hospitalization needs during an outpatient rehabilitation program for severe CAO. *Chest*. 1976;70:606-610.

34. Bebout DE, Hodgkin JE, Zorn EG, et al. Clinical and physiological outcomes of a university-hospital pulmonary rehabilitation program. *Respir Care*. 1983;23:1468-1473.

35. Continuous or nocturnal oxygen therapy in hypoxemic chronic obstructive lung disease: a clinical trial. *Am Inter Med*. 1980;93:391-398.

36. Bunch D. Pulmonary rehabilitation: the next ten years. *AARC Times*. 1988;12(3):54.

Chapter 2

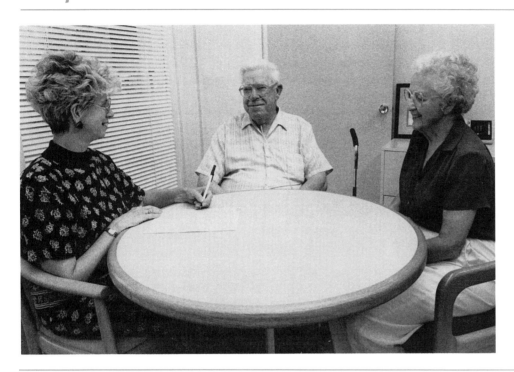

Selection and Team Assessment of the Pulmonary Rehabilitation Candidate

The specific criteria for accepting a patient into a pulmonary rehabilitation program may vary depending upon the individual patient goals and the program itself.[1] Written criteria help facilitate interactions with third-party payors and potential patients. Exceptions and variations to usual guidelines should be documented carefully, with appropriate explanations. A comprehensive rehabilitation program may be adapted for any individual with pulmonary disease. Physical or other disabilities do not necessarily exclude a prospective candidate. Table 2.1 lists conditions appropriate for pulmonary rehabilitation.

Patient selection criteria help facilitate interactions with third-party payors and potential patients.

Table 2.1 Conditions Appropriate for Pulmonary Rehabilitation

Obstructive pulmonary disease
  Chronic obstructive pulmonary disease (COPD)
  Asthma
  Asthmatic bronchitis
  Chronic bronchitis
  Emphysema
  Bronchiectasis
  Cystic fibrosis

Restrictive pulmonary disease
  Interstitial fibrosis
  Rheumatoid pulmonary disease
  Collagen vascular lung disorders
  Pneumoconiosis
  Sarcoidosis
  Kyphoscoliosis
  Rheumatoid spondylitis
  Severe obesity
  Poliomyelitis

Other conditions
  Pulmonary vascular diseases
  Lung resection
  Lung transplantation
  Occupational/environmental lung diseases

Note. Reprinted with permission from "Organization and Management of a Pulmonary Rehabilitation Program" by L. Beytas and G.L. Connors. In *Pulmonary Rehabilitation: Guidelines to Success* (2nd ed.) by J.E. Hodgkin, G.L. Connors, and C.W. Bell (Eds.). Copyright 1992 by J.B. Lippincott.

Patient Selection

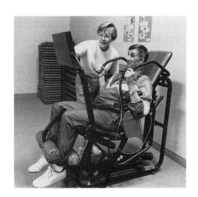

Most comprehensive programs enroll patients who are in a stable phase of their disease. In some instances, rehabilitation may be implemented during ventilator-assisted care and recovery from an acute illness. Pulmonary function testing is essential in detecting, confirming, and staging many pulmonary diseases. See Table 2.2 for the indications for pulmonary function testing. Standard criteria appropriate for each type of pulmonary disease should be used in detecting abnormalities in pulmonary function.[2,3] See Table 2.3, which looks at the physiological determinants of lung disease characterized by the major symptoms and patterns of airflow obstruction (trapping and residual volume, hyperinflation, and diffusion). Then refer to Table 2.4, which details the patterns of pulmonary function abnormalities in obstructive, restrictive, and mixed pulmonary disease compared with normal function.

Table 2.2 Indications for Pulmonary Function Tests

Identify the high risk smoker	Determine the cause of dyspnea
Early detection of lung disease	Evaluate the risk of postoperative complications
Follow the course of lung disease	Evaluate effects of occupational exposures
Measure therapy effectiveness	Determine degree of impairment (medicolegal)

Note. Reprinted with permission from ''Pulmonary Function Tests'' by P.L. Enright and J.E. Hodgkin. In *Respiratory Care: A Guide to Clinical Practice* (3rd ed.) (p. 158) by G.G. Burton, J.E. Hodgkin, and J.J. Ward (Eds.). Copyright 1991 by J.B. Lippincott.

Table 2.3 Physiological Determinants of Diseases Characterized by Acute and Chronic Airflow Obstruction

Disease	Major symptoms complex	Pattern of airflow obstruction (FEV_1)	Trapping and residual volume	Hyperinflation	Diffusion
Intermittent asthma	Acute wheezing, dyspnea, with variable cough	Reversible airflow obstruction	Mild, intermittent	Transient	Normal
Asthmatic and chronic bronchitis	Chronic cough, wheeze, with variable degrees of dyspnea	Partly reversible or irreversible airflow obstruction	Moderate, partly reversible	Mild to moderate	Normal and slightly reduced
Emphysema	Dyspnea, variable cough and wheeze	Irreversible airflow obstruction, progressive impairment	Moderate to marked, progressive	Moderate to marked	Reduced
COPD, advanced	Elements of asthma, chronic bronchitis, and emphysema—mostly owing to emphysema and irreversible changes in the conducting airways				

Note. Reprinted with permission from ''Definitions of Airflow Disorders and Implications for Therapy'' by T.L. Petty. In *Respiratory Care: A Guide to Clinical Practice* (3rd ed.) (p. 934) by G.G. Burton, J.E. Hodgkin, and J.J. Ward (Eds.). Copyright 1991 by J.B. Lippincott.

Table 2.4 Patterns of Pulmonary Function Abnormality

	Normal	Obstruction	Restriction	Mixed
FEV_1/FVC	≥90% predicted	Low	Normal to high	Low
FEV_1	≥80% predicted	Low	Low	Low
FVC	≥80% predicted	Normal to low	Low	Low
TLC	80%-120% predicted	Normal to high	Low	Normal to low
RV/TLC	25%-40%	High	Normal	High

Note. Reprinted with permission from ''Pulmonary Function Tests'' by P.L. Enright and J.E. Hodgkin. In *Respiratory Care: A Guide to Clinical Practice* (3rd ed.) (p. 178) by G.G. Burton, J.E. Hodgkin, and J.J. Ward (Eds.). Copyright 1991 by J.B. Lippincott.

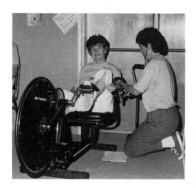

Although pulmonary function testing is very helpful in assessing patients for rehabilitation, specific criteria for impairment of pulmonary function should not be used alone in establishing eligibility for such programs. The most important element should be a careful assessment of the effects of the disease on the patient's quality of life. Factors such as reduction in physical activity, occupational performance, independence in activities of daily living, and use of medical resources should be evaluated and documented. Similar to the principles of disability evaluation for patients with pulmonary disease, an important criterion for eligibility should be whether the disease is causing any limitations for the patient, not just whether the disease is present.[4] See Appendix A, pp. 76-78, for further guidelines on patient evaluation. See Table 2.5 for a list of criteria for selecting patients for rehabilitation.

Table 2.5   Criteria to Be Evaluated in Selecting a Patient for Pulmonary Rehabilitation*

Disease effect on patient's quality of life
Reduction in physical activity
Changes in occupational performance
Dependence vs. independence in activities of daily living
Disease effect on the patient's psychosocial status (i.e., anxiety, depression, etc.)
Use of medical resources (i.e., hospitalizations, emergency room visits, etc.)
Presence of other medical problems
Pulmonary function assessment
Smoking history
Patient motivation
Patient commitment to time and active program participation
Patient transportation needs
Financial resources
Patient's background

*Any patient with impairment because of lung disease and who is motivated should be a candidate for pulmonary rehabilitation.
Note. Reprinted with permission from "Organization and Management of a Pulmonary Rehabilitation Program" by L. Beytas and G.L. Connors. In *Pulmonary Rehabilitation: Guidelines to Success* (2nd ed.) by J.E. Hodgkin, G.L. Connors, and C.W. Bell (Eds.). Copyright 1992 by J.B. Lippincott.

Pulmonary rehabilitation programs emphasize active patient involvement and responsibility for their own health care. Therefore, in selecting patients, it is important to assess and document, during the initial interview, a patient's understanding of, interest in, and willingness to actively participate in a comprehensive care program, because these affect outcomes. The documentation may be in the form of a questionnaire or an assessment form developed by the program. See Figure 2.1 for an example of a pulmonary rehabilitation evaluation form.

Current smoking status has been used by some in accepting or denying a patient's entrance into a rehabilitation program. Complete smoking cessation may not be necessary for patients entering a program, but it should be addressed as an important goal for these patients.

Patients enrolling in a comprehensive program should be capable of committing the time, effort, and attention necessary to achieve their

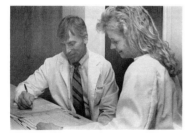

Figure 2.1
Pulmonary Rehabilitation Evaluation Form

Primary diagnosis: _____

_____

_____

Chief complaint: _____

_____

_____

Medical history

_____ Cardiac complications

_____ Hypertension

_____ Diabetes

_____ GI problems

_____ Reflux/hiatal hernia

_____ Orthopedic problems

_____ PND/sinus problems

_____ Vision/hearing

_____ Childhood illnesses

_____ Other _____

Symptoms

Y N Cough Frequency _____

Y N Sputum
         Volume _____ Color _____
         Viscosity _____ Frequency _____

Y N Wheeze
         Onset/cause _____

Y N Fluid retention
         Where _____ When _____

Y N Dyspnea
         Onset/cause _____

Y N Sleeping problems # hours _____

Y N Extra pillows # _____

Dyspnea index (circle one)

Class 1: If SOB, consistent with activity

Class 2: SOB climbing hills or stairs

Class 3: Can walk at own pace but not at normal pace without SOB

Class 4: SOB walking 100 yds on level ground, dressing, or talking

Allergies

Food: _____

Medications: _____

Others: _____

Occupation

Occupation _____

Retirement/disability date _____

Occupational exposures:

_____ Farm/ranch   _____ Pottery

_____ Welding   _____ Gas/fumes

_____ Mines/foundry   _____ Chemicals

_____ Sandblasting   _____ Dust

_____ Quarry   _____ Asbestos

Respiratory infections/hospitalizations

_____ Infections/year
         Antibiotic use: _____

_____ Hospitalizations/year
         When: _____
         Problem: _____

Vaccines: Flu _____ (year)
          Pneumonia _____ (year)

Y N Aware of warning signals?

Smoking history

Y N Quit date _____
         _____ Packs _____ Years

Y N Secondhand smoke

Breathing retraining

Y N Pursed-lip breathing

Y N Diaphragm breathing

Y N Accessory muscle use

Objective

B/P _____   Br Sds _____

HR _____   Edema _____

RR _____   Other _____

(continued)

Figure 2.1 *(continued)*

Metered dose inhalers (MDI)

MDI #1 _____

   Prescription _____

MDI #2 _____

   Prescription _____

MDI #3 _____

   Prescription _____

MDI #4 _____

   Prescription _____

Y   N   Needs spacer

Y   N   Needs training

Oral medications

_____   _____

_____   _____

_____   _____

Stress management

Stressors: _____

_____

Relaxation techniques: _____

Current exercise program: _____

Leisure activities: _____

_____

Assessment

1. Understanding of diagnosis _____

2. Personal goals _____

   _____

3. _____

Plan

1. _____

2. _____

3. _____

Aerosol therapy

Y   N   Hand-held nebulizer

Vendor: _____

Medication: Type   Dose

_____

_____

_____

Frequency prescribed vs. use: _____

Oxygen therapy

Y   N   Oxygen therapy

Y   N   Needs training

System/Vendor: _____

Fluid intake   (Glasses/day):

_____ Water   _____ Beer

_____ Soda   _____ Hard liquor

_____ Wine   _____ Coffee

_____ Juice   _____ Tea

Nutrition

Appetite: _____

Diet: _____

Restaurants/week: _____

Salt use (restriction): _____

Vitamins: _____

_____   _____

Staff   Date

goals. Concurrent diseases or conditions that may interfere with the rehabilitation process should be recognized, corrected, or stabilized before the patient enters the program. Permanent or temporary conditions that may be considered contraindications to pulmonary rehabilitation include, but are not limited to, the conditions listed in Table 2.6.

Table 2.6 Permanent or Temporary Conditions That May Be Considered Contraindications To Pulmonary Rehabilitation

Severe psychiatric disturbance
  Dementia
  Organic brain syndrome

Significant or unstable medical conditions
  Congestive heart failure
  Acute cor pulmonale
  Substance abuse
  Significant liver dysfunction
  Metastatic cancer
  Disabling stroke

Note. Reprinted with permission from "Organization and Management of a Pulmonary Rehabilitation Program" by L. Beytas and G.L. Connors. In *Pulmonary Rehabilitation: Guidelines to Success* (2nd ed.) by J.E. Hodgkin, G.L. Connors, and C.W. Bell (Eds.). Copyright 1992 by J.B. Lippincott.

Other issues to be addressed with the future rehabilitation patient should include financial considerations and transportation.

It is essential to discuss the patient's financial ability to meet the expenses of the program before he or she is accepted into the program. Third-party payors should be contacted to determine if the rehabilitation program is covered and to what extent. The patient is then able to determine if he or she will be able to bear the additional costs. Verbal and written information regarding cost and coverage is critical prior to admission to the program rather than when the first bill arrives.

Transportation is another issue that is important to discuss prior to entering the program. Patients must have a means of getting to the program. If patients are independent and not debilitated, they may drive themselves. Family members may provide the transportation or they may have to rely on public transit. Local and regional telephone books, in their yellow or blue pages, have transportation assistance information from state and federal agencies listed under the disabled, handicapped, and aging headings.

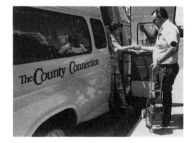

Some programs assist the patient in addressing the insurance and transportation issues; other programs make it the responsibility of the patient. If the latter is the case, then it is important to describe who, what, when, and how in written form for the patient. Have the patient do all of the investigation before he or she begins the program.

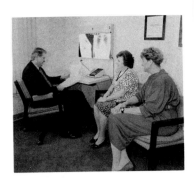

The patient assessment should focus on the following: medical history, physical assessment, psychosocial issues, nutritional status, exercise ability, and activities of daily living.

A number of medical facilities have a well-developed Social Work Department. The social work staff may assist patients with questions such as medical assistance, transportation, and community support networks. This department should be an integral part of the pulmonary rehabilitation team.

Patient Assessment

A thorough review of the patient's general medical history and records is the foundation for the assessment of a patient for pulmonary rehabilitation. Program staff should obtain available records from the patient's primary source of medical care. An in-depth interview with the patient and family or significant others is necessary to establish appropriate individual patient goals for the program. This initial assessment should include the hobbies, psychosocial, and vocational areas (review Figure 2.1 on pages 15-16). Questionnaires or forms may be used to assess symptoms such as dyspnea, cough, sputum production, wheezing, edema, depression, and specific problems in activities of daily living. The results of the initial evaluations are reviewed with other team members. Additional diagnostic evaluation or treatment may then be arranged, as indicated.

The initial assessment should pay particular attention to the patient's medical history, including symptoms; physical assessment; psychosocial, nutritional, and exercise tolerance; and the patient's ability to carry out activities of daily living.[5,6]

Symptoms

Documenting the patient's stated symptoms during the initial evaluation is critical. It is important to cover the onset; location; quality; quantity; frequency; duration; aggravating, alleviating, and associated factors; and the cause of each symptom when and where applicable. The following lists the most common symptoms reported by pulmonary patients.

- Dyspnea
- Cough
- Sputum production
- Wheezing
- Hemoptysis
- Edema
- Chest pain

Pertinent Medical History

A thorough evaluation of prior medical history of new patients entering the program must cover many areas. An assessment may be in the form of a self-report questionnaire sent to the patient to complete prior to the initial interview or given immediately before the interview begins. It is essential to evaluate medical conditions that often are found in the "other" category. These conditions, although not pulmonary in nature, may have a direct bearing on lung health. "Other" categories to pay particular attention to are gastrointestinal, nasal/sinus, cardiovascular, neurological, and musculoskeletal. The following lists specifics regarding the information to be gathered for a complete medical history.

- Smoking history
- Occupational and environmental exposure to pulmonary irritants[7]
- Recreational/hobby exposure to pulmonary irritants
- Alcohol history
- Medications
- Childhood pulmonary problems
- Family history of pulmonary diseases
- Other medical problems including[8,9]:

  - Gastroesophageal reflux with chronic aspiration
  - Hiatal hernia
  - Sinusitis/rhinitis
  - Cardiovascular disease
  - Sleep disturbances
  - Neuromuscular and orthopedic impairment

Physical Assessment

In the preliminary screening, physical assessment includes measuring and evaluating the basic vital signs. Depending on the needs of the patient and the requirements of the program, the following is a list of common physical assessment items.

- Blood pressure
- Heart rate
- Respiratory rate
- Breath sounds
- Use of accessory muscles
- Edema
- Jugular venous pressure to assess right heart function

Psychosocial Assessment

Psychosocial assessment is covered in chapter 5. In general, psychosocial evaluation and treatment should be integrated into every component of pulmonary rehabilitation from assessment through follow-up.[10]

Nutritional Assessment

A nutritional evaluation for the pulmonary-impaired patient is important.[11] Individual patient goals may include fluid intake for secretion management, sodium reduction, weight loss for the overweight patient (to decrease the work of breathing), or weight gain for the underweight patient. In fact, a reduced body weight independent of the patient's FEV_1 is an important predictor of survival.[12] The chronic pulmonary patient has an increased energy expenditure to breathe, which results in increased caloric needs.[13] Problems of maintaining adequate nutrition are present in 40% to 60% of patients with COPD.[14] The extent of the nutritional assessment depends upon the patient's needs.

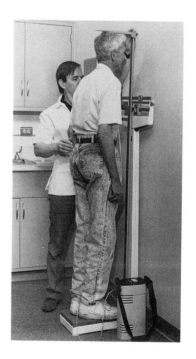

Exercise Assessment

The safety of an exercise training program and an appropriate exercise prescription is determined by the thoroughness of the initial

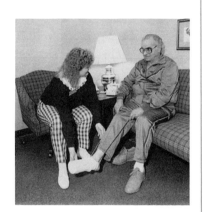

exercise assessment. An assessment must be done to evaluate the patient's exercise tolerance, hypoxemia, and whether supplemental oxygen is required during exercise. Additionally, the assessment should include an evaluation of cardiac function. Chapter 4 discusses a variety of exercise testing procedures and protocols that may be used.

Once the exercise assessment is completed, the exercise program is developed for the pulmonary-impaired patient to avoid becoming a "respiratory cripple." Too often, increased shortness of breath results in decreased activity, leading to worsening muscle weakness and a downhill cycle. An increase in work capacity along with an enhanced sense of well-being have been documented in pulmonary patients who participate in an exercise training program[15-19] (see chapter 4).

Activities of Daily Living Assessment

The patient's ability to function independently in activities of daily living (ADL), leisure activities, and sexual performance should be assessed. Dyspnea often leads to a decreased ability and willingness to perform daily activities independently. Through the ADL assessment, the need for energy conservation techniques, proper breathing training with daily activities, and adaptive equipment should be evaluated. An occupational therapist (or other allied health professional) may perform the ADL assessment, and a recreational therapist (or other allied health professional) may help to evaluate the patient's leisure impairment. An upper extremity evaluation and an assessment of functional-tasks performance and the work environment's demands, if applicable, should also be performed.

Role of Sexuality

The patient's sexual function or dysfunction is a critical area to be assessed. Understanding the patient's fears, concerns, and previous patterns of sexual activity will help to plan for counseling. The reaction of the significant other to the disease and its effect on mutual sexual function is important in this area. Table 2.7 provides an assessment tool for the health care professional to follow when evaluating the patient's sexual function—past, present, and future. Utilization of this baseline information will help determine counseling needs.

Medical Testing

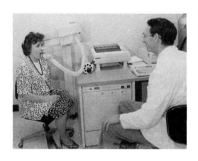

In addition to reviewing recent diagnostic test results, program staff should obtain additional laboratory tests per physician order as necessary to complete the evaluation and plan an individualized treatment program.[20] It is important to compare previous test results with current test results in assessing the patient's status. The minimum tests suggested during the initial evaluation of a rehabilitation candidate are listed in Table 2.8.

Additional laboratory tests may be appropriate as a result of the thorough initial assessment. Other tests that may be appropriate for selected patients are presented in Table 2.9.

**Table 2.7 Assessment of the Chronic Pulmonary Patient
With Sexual Dysfunction**

Assessment	Rationale
Previous patterns of sexual activity a. Partner availability b. Types of sexual behaviors c. Frequency and duration d. Usual time of day e. Positions favored and initiator	Obtain baseline information needed to assess needs and individualize counseling For it to be effective, counseling must take into account personal preferences and expectations for the relationship
Past experience with shortness of breath during intercourse and/or sexual stimulation (severity and response)	Shortness of breath common experience for pulmonary patients, which can lead to increased anxiety in the patient and partner
History of sexual difficulty prior to the pulmonary illness a. Kind and frequency b. Stressful circumstances c. Medications and alcohol d. Presence of disease e. Presence of ''wet dreams'' and ''morning erections''	Determine if the current problem is one of organic or of psychogenic dysfunction
Psychosocial data a. Attitudes toward sex and sexuality b. Reaction of patient and sex partner to illness	Myths and misconceptions can be a cause of sexual difficulties

Note. Adapted with permission from ''Areas of Assessment for Sexual Dysfunction in Post Coronary Patients'' by C. Scalzi and K. Dracup, 1978, *Heart & Lung,* **7**(5), p. 843. Copyright 1978 by Mosby-Year Book, Inc.

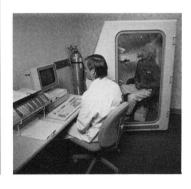

Table 2.8 Suggested Tests During Initial Evaluation of a Pulmonary Rehabilitation Candidate

Spirometry pre/post bronchodilator Lung volumes Diffusing capacity Resting arterial blood gas Chest radiograph Resting electrocardiogram	Exercise test with cutaneous oximetry and/or arterial blood gas (simple or modified test such as 6- or 12-minute walk, Master's step, calibrated cycle ergometer, or motorized treadmill) Complete blood count Basic blood chemistry panel

Note. It is acceptable to not repeat these tests if done within the 3 months prior to entering the pulmonary rehabilitation program or as determined by the pulmonary rehabilitation medical director.

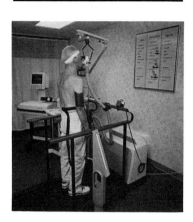

Table 2.9   Other Tests to Consider for Selected Patients

Maximal voluntary ventilation

Maximal inspiratory and expiratory pressures

Theophylline level, when applicable

Pulmonary exercise stress test (metabolic study) with continuous ECG monitoring

Postexercise spirometry

Bronchial challenge

Cardiovascular tests (e.g., holter monitor, echocardiogram, thallium exercise stress test)

Polysomnography

Sinus X rays

Upper gastrointestinal series

Skin tests

Conclusion

Initial assessment is a crucial component of comprehensive pulmonary rehabilitation. Training alone or in conjunction with exercise is not pulmonary rehabilitation unless a thorough initial assessment is accomplished. In fact, for third-party reimbursement, a deficit and need for treatment must be determined and documented. The team approach does not mean every patient needs to be assessed by every team member; however, when the patient's deficits are determined, they must be addressed. An individualized rehabilitation program for the pulmonary-impaired patient is accomplished only after a thorough assessment.

References

1. Hodge-Hilton T, Herrmann D, Hills R, Feenstra L, Archibald C. Initial evaluation of the pulmonary rehabilitation candidate. In: Hodgkin JE, Zorn EG, Connors GL, eds. *Pulmonary Rehabilitation: Guidelines to Success*. Boston, Mass: Butterworth; 1984;4:27-43.
2. Official statement of the American Thoracic Society. Standards for the diagnosis and care of patients with chronic obstructive pulmonary disease (COPD) and asthma. *Am Rev Respir Dis*. 1987;136(1):225.
3. George RB, Anderson WM. Laboratory evaluation of patients with COPD. In: Hodgkin JE, Petty TL, eds. *Chronic Obstructive Pulmonary Disease: Current Concepts*. Philadelphia, PA: WB Saunders; 1987:36-63.
4. American Thoracic Society. Evaluation of impairment/disability secondary to respiratory disorders. *Am Rev Respir Dis*. 1986;133:1205-1209.

5. Connors GL, Hodgkin JE. Pulmonary rehabilitation. In: Burton GG, Hodgkin JE, Ward JJ, eds. *Respiratory Care: A Guide to Clinical Practice*. 3rd ed. Philadelphia, PA: JB Lippincott; 1991:655.

6. Wilkins RL, Hodgkin JE. History and physical examination of the respiratory patient. In: Burton GG, Hodgkin JE, Ward JJ, eds. *Respiratory Care—A Guide to Clinical Practice*. 3rd ed. Philadelphia, PA: JB Lippincott; 1991:211.

7. Hodgkin JE, Abbey DE, Euler GL, Magie AR. COPD prevalence in nonsmokers in high and low photochemical air pollution areas. *Chest*. 1984;86(6):830-838.

8. Branscomb BV. Aggravating factors and coexisting disorders. In: Hodgkin JE, Petty TL, eds. *Chronic Obstructive Pulmonary Disease: Current Concepts*. Philadelphia, PA: WB Saunders; 1987:183.

9. Connors GL, Hodgkin JE, Asmus RM. A careful assessment is crucial to successful pulmonary rehabilitation. *J Cardiopul Rehab*. 1988;8(11):435-438.

10. Burke P, Meyer V, Kocoshis S, et al. Depression and anxiety in pediatric inflammatory bowel disease and cystic fibrosis. *J Am Acad Child Adolesc Psychiatry*. 1989;28:948-951.

11. Donahoe M, Rogers RM. Nutritional assessment and support in chronic obstructive pulmonary disease. *Clinics in Chest Medicine*. 1990;11(3):487-504.

12. Wilson DO, Rogers RM, Wright EC, Anthonisen NR. Body weight in chronic obstructive pulmonary disease. The National Institutes of Health intermittent positive-pressure breathing trial. *Am Rev Respir Dis*. 1989;139:1435-1438.

13. Branson RD, Hurst JM. Nutrition and respiratory function: food for thought. *Resp Care*. 1988;33(2):89-92. Editorial.

14. Rhodes ML. General principles of care. In: Hodgkin JE, Petty TL, eds. *Chronic Obstructive Pulmonary Disease: Current Concepts*. Philadelphia, PA: WB Saunders; 1987.

15. Braun NMT, Rochester DF. Respiratory muscle strength in obstructive lung disease. *Am Rev Respir Dis*. 1977;115:91.

16. Sharp JT, Danon J, Druz WS, et al. Respiratory muscle function in patients with chronic obstructive pulmonary disease: its relationship to disability and to respiratory therapy. *Am Rev Respir Dis*. 1974; 100:154.

17. Pierce AK, Taylor HF, Archer RK, et al. Responses to exercise training in patients with emphysema. *Arch Intern Med*. 1964;113:28.

18. Orenstein DM, Franklin BA, Doershuk CF, et al. Exercise conditioning and cardiopulmonary fitness in cystic fibrosis. The effects of a three-month supervised running program. *Chest*. 1981;80:392-398.

19. Orenstein DM, Henke KG, Ceruz FJ. Exercise and cystic fibrosis. *Physician Sports Med*. 1983;11:57-62.

20. Enright PL, Hodgkin JE. Pulmonary function tests. In: Burton GG, Hodgkin JE, Ward JJ, eds. *Respiratory Care—A Guide to Clinical Practice*. 3rd ed. Philadelphia, PA: JB Lippincott; 1991:157.

Chapter 3

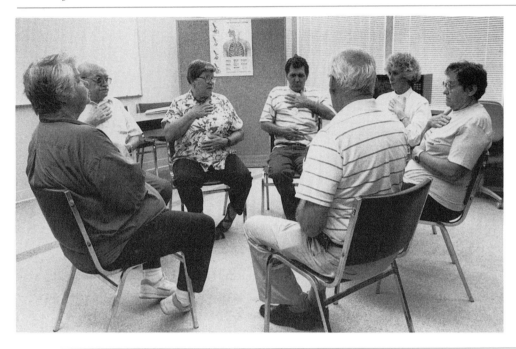

Patient Training

To achieve the goals of pulmonary rehabilitation, both the patient and the significant other(s) must understand the patient's underlying pulmonary disorder and principles of management.[1] The objective of the training program should be to encourage patients to make behavioral changes that will lead to improved health by making them active participants in their own health care.[2-4] Each adult learner will have an individualized approach to accepting new information based on her or his previous life experiences.[5] Educators of adults should remain aware that these individuals have accumulated a vast reservoir of experiences. This experiential background is a rich resource to facilitate the learning process.[6] Many times experiences need the benefit of professional interpretation and explanation to enhance their value.

New information is most often acquired in three ways—through auditory, visual, and kinesthetic (doing) processes—but each individual usually gains new information from one learning process more often and more effectively than from the others.[7] Determining the adult learner's primary learning style can assist the educator in enhancing the patient's learning. In fact, when developing the training program, the team members may want to use each of the processes to improve the retention of the newly learned material. Repetition, straightforwardness, and respecting the patient are important aspects of achieving

> The training program should encourage patients to make behavioral changes that will lead to improved health.

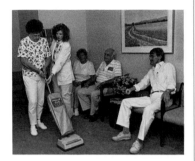

successful educational training. Because the development of pulmonary disease is such a long-term process, many of the patients entering pulmonary rehabilitation are middle-aged or older. As a result, these patients may have been removed from the educational setting for many years and may not be involved in utilizing learning and retention skills. Figure 3.1 depicts a scale of learning that demonstrates the ability to increase information retention through use of each of the senses. Research with this tool has demonstrated that utilization of the senses (seeing, hearing, touching, etc.) in learning material produces greater retention. The expected outcome in developing a personalized pulmonary program for each patient is: What the patient needs to know is not only learned but also applied. Additionally, the reading level of the average American adult is between Grades 6 and 8; therefore, reading materials should be written accordingly.

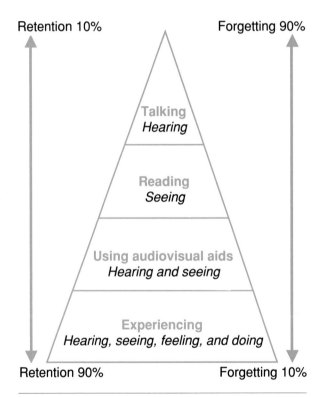

Figure 3.1   The scale of learning.

Note. Reprinted with permission from "Education of Patients and Their Families" by J.W. Hopp and S.E. Maddox. In *Pulmonary Rehabilitation: Guidelines to Success* (p. 55) by J.E. Hodgkin, E.G. Zorn, and G.L. Connors (Eds.). Copyright 1984 by J.E. Hodgkin.

The training program covers these various areas: self-assessment, bronchial hygiene, activities of daily living, medications, respiratory modalities, and psychosocial interventions.

The specific content covered will depend upon the *individualized goals* for the patient. The training sessions may be conducted by professionals from any of the disciplines on the rehabilitation team.

Any or all of the following topics may be included in a typical program, depending upon the patient's individual needs.

Self-Assessment

A primary objective of pulmonary rehabilitation is to assist the patient in achieving his or her optimum level of function. The patient's educational and self-assessment needs are determined during the initial evaluation and reassessment. Figure 3.2 and Tables 3.1 and 3.2 demonstrate the types of components that may be covered when helping patients evaluate their responses to shortness of breath, alcohol intake, or medications. For example, Figure 3.2 is a tool that may facilitate the patient's understanding of nutrition in good health and the process by which food desirability decreases as respiratory symptoms increase. Tables 3.1 and 3.2 are teaching tools to increase understanding of the role alcohol and medications may have on symptoms and nutritional status. The following list names additional areas that should be covered as indicated by patient needs. In all cases it is important to individualize the training and to insure that the patient knows how to assess his or her needs.

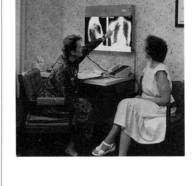

- Anatomy and physiology of the respiratory system
- Respiratory disease process
- Description and interpretation of medical tests
- Principles of exercise and physical fitness
- Home exercise prescription
- Nutrition and the lungs (see Figure 3.2, Table 3.1, and Table 3.2)
- Self-assessment and symptom management
- Warning signs of an infection
- Other areas of self-assessment based upon the ongoing patient assessment

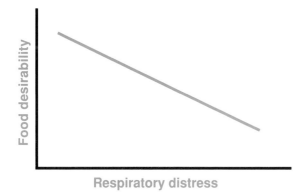

Figure 3.2   There is an inverse relationship between food desirability and respiratory distress. As the level of respiratory distress increases, the chances of optimal nutrition decrease. At some point invasive intervention (tube feedings or parenteral nutrition) may be necessary.

Note. Reprinted with permission from "Nutrition and the Pulmonary Patient" by J.A. Peters, K. Burke, and D. White. In *Pulmonary Rehabilitation: Guidelines to Success* (p. 265) by J.E. Hodgkin, E.G. Zorn, and G.L. Connors (Eds.). Copyright 1984 by J.E. Hodgkin.

Table 3.1 Ingestion of Alcohol as It Relates to Lung Disease

Dehydrates cells
Alcohol metabolism unrelated to energy needs
Increases requirements for other nutrients
Decreases FVC
Decreases FEV_1
Decreases DLCO
Induces bronchoconstriction
Impairs clearance of bacteria from lungs
Impairs function of type II alveolar cells
Alters $\dot{V}/\dot{Q}$ matchup in lung
Increases metabolic acidosis
Interacts with adenylate cyclase
Enhances likelihood of sleep apnea

Note. Reprinted with permission from ''Nutrition and the Pulmonary Patient'' by J.A. Peters, K. Burke, and D. White. In *Pulmonary Rehabilitation: Guidelines to Success* (p. 271) by J.E. Hodgkin, E.G. Zorn, and G.L. Connors (Eds.). Copyright 1984 by J.E. Hodgkin.

Table 3.2 Effects of Selected Medications on Nutritional Status and Appetite

Medication	Nutritional effect	Possible GI effects
Antacids	Aluminum hydroxide gel increases phosphate excretion. Edema may result from high sodium. Decreased absorption of iron and vitamin B_1	May see constipation, diarrhea, steatorrhea
Antihypertensives	May cause vitamin B_6 depletion	Anorexia, nausea, vomiting, diarrhea
Antibiotics	Protein, calcium, magnesium, iron, vitamins K, B_{12}, amino acid absorption, and protein synthesis may be inhibited during long-duration therapy. Chloramphenicol causes lactose malabsorption. Tetracycline binds to calcium. Neomycin decreases absorption of fats and fat soluble vitamins, and bile salts. Isoniazid interferes with B_6 metabolism, thus niacin and tryptophan metabolism affected	Diarrhea, steatorrhea, nausea, vomiting, stomatitis, decreased taste acuity, anorexia
Antiflammatory agents	Salicylates and indomethacin increase urinary excretion of vitamin C. Phenylbutazone decreases absorption of folic acid	GI irritation
Analgesics	Morphine and other narcotics may cause decreased gastric and pancreatic secretions, decreased peristalsis. ASA can increase GI blood loss	Constipation, diarrhea, vomiting, nausea, blood loss, decreased appetite
Anticonvulsants and sedatives	Barbiturates and hydantoins may decrease folate and vitamin D. Barbiturates may decrease B_{12} absorption. Glutethimide may decrease folate levels	Hyperplasia of gums, constipation, GI irritation, nausea, vomiting
Cardiac glycosides	Depleted potassium may cause digitalis toxicity. Increased serum calcium levels may produce arrhythmias. Digitoxin decreases glucose absorption	Appetite may be depressed. GI irritation may be seen, nausea, vomiting

Medication	Nutritional effect	Possible GI effects
Corticosteroids	Cortisone may accelerate vitamin D metabolism, which may accelerate bone loss. Prednisone may increase vitamin B_6 requirement. May increase zinc, potassium, and magnesium excretion. Glucose tolerance may be decreased. Fat mobilization and/or fatty liver may occur	May be increased appetite due to euphoria. May see either decrease or increase in gastric secretion
Diuretics	Thiazides may increase uric acid levels and decrease glucose tolerance. Increased sodium and potassium loss. May also increase urinary calcium, zinc, magnesium, and other electrolyte losses. Excessive loss of potassium in cardiac patients receiving digitalis may precipitate toxicity. Low-sodium and low-potassium diets may result in hyponaturemia or hypokalemia. Spironolactone reduces potassium excretion and may result in hyperkalemia	GI irritation, nausea, vomiting, diarrhea, abdominal pain
Cathartics, laxatives	Protein-losing enteropathy may result from excessive use. Potassium, magnesium, calcium, sodium, and fluid losses may occur. Malabsorption is often seen. Mineral oil causes decreased absorption of fat soluble vitamins (A, D, E, K). Milk of magnesia decreases absorption of fat and phosphates. Phenolphthalein results in decreased absorption of vitamin D and calcium	Abdominal cramps, steatorrhea
Tranquilizers	Edema may occur due to sodium	May increase appetite and decrease taste acuity. May cause dry mouth, constipation, diarrhea
Oral contraceptives	May cause increased vitamin B_6 and riboflavin requirement, decreased folate absorption. May increase serum copper, hemoglobin, plasma vitamin A levels. May decrease leucocyte, vitamin C, and plasma B_{12} levels. Increase in calcium absorption	Constipation or diarrhea may be seen
Alcohol	Decreased absorption and utilization of folates. Increased need and decreased absorption of thiamine. Decreased conversion of vitamin B_6 to active form. Decreased absorption of zinc and magnesium	Increased gastric acid secretion. GI irritation and diarrhea may occur with high intake
Theophylline	May act as a diuretic causing increased loss of sodium and potassium	GI distress, increased GI secretion, nausea, vomiting
Oral hypoglycemic agents	May cause decreased vitamin B_{12} absorption	GI distress, nausea, vomiting
Potassium chloride	May decrease vitamin B_{12} absorption	May cause GI distress
Sodium chloride (aerosolized saline)	May increase sodium levels	None

Note. Reprinted with permission from ''Nutrition and the Pulmonary Patient'' by J.A. Peters, K. Burke, and D. White. In *Pulmonary Rehabilitation: Guidelines to Success* (p. 272-273) by J.E. Hodgkin, E.G. Zorn, and G.L. Connors (Eds.). Copyright 1984 by J.E. Hodgkin.

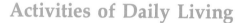

Bronchial Hygiene

Good bronchial hygiene is a daily requirement for the pulmonary patient to ensure optimum airflow. The pulmonary rehabilitation team should teach the individual to understand his or her bronchial hygiene needs and how to assess such things as the work of breathing, utilization of accessory muscles, cough technique, and shortness of breath. The following lists areas that should be covered with each patient as determined by the patient's needs.

- Breathing retraining, including pursed-lip[8] and diaphragmatic breathing
- Postural drainage therapy (PDT), including positioning and percussion[9,10]
- Cough techniques[11,12]
- Positive expiratory pressure (PEP)
- Autogenic drainage
- Other areas of bronchial hygiene based upon the ongoing patient assessment

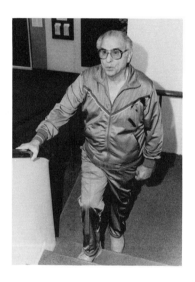

Activities of Daily Living

Independence in activities of daily living is a primary goal for the pulmonary patient. The initial assessment should include an evaluation of ADL and self-care abilities. Deficiencies should be addressed and may include but are not limited to those areas listed here. Sexual activities are often ignored by health professionals, however, it is essential to evaluate this area. Table 3.3 presents the P LI SS IT model, which is a tool for the pulmonary rehabilitation team member to use in addressing these sensitive issues. The patient may not need assistance in this area, or the patient may just need permission to be sexually intimate. Specific suggestions may be required or there may be a need for intensive therapy through referral to a counselor or sex therapist.

     Many other areas are included in ADL and should be covered as determined by each patient's needs.

- Time and energy conservation techniques
- Leisure-time activities[13]
- Panic control and relaxation
- Sexuality (see Table 3.3)
- Travel recommendations for lung patients[14,15]
- Community resources
- Vocational retraining[16]
- Other areas of activities of daily living based upon the ongoing patient assessment

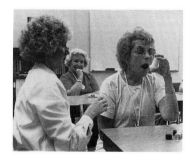

Medications[17-19]

Training in the use, side effects, and role of medications in the treatment and prevention of lung impairment is a critical area for pulmonary patients. A major outcome measure of patient responsibility in self-care is adherence and compliance to the medication regimen. There

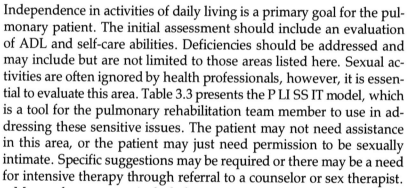

Table 3.3 The P LI SS IT Model

P — Giving Permission

Objective: Provide validation and reassurance that it is permissible to have sexual concerns and feelings, and to engage in sexual behavior.

Guidelines: (1) Include questions on sexual functioning during the initial interview along with other activities of daily living. (2) Ask open-ended questions. (3) Convey a pleasure-based rather than a performance-based view of sexuality. (4) Listen carefully for ''implied messages.'' (5) Encourage the couple to explore their own sexual and sensual potentials. (6) Utilize terminology familiar to the patient, and avoid labels. (7) Encourage further exploration of all indirect and partial responses.

LI — Providing Limited Information

Objective: Respond to the patient's questions with factual information.

Guidelines: (1) Distinguish between organic and psychogenic impotence. (2) Discuss the expected sexual changes with aging. (3) Discuss the energy requirements during intercourse, and reassure the patient that some shortness of breath is not necessarily a sign of danger. (4) Caution the patient regarding the possible effects of increasing dosage of medication, and alcohol intake, on sexual functioning.

SS — Giving Specific Suggestions

Objective: Assist the patient in the alleviation or reduction of stated sexual difficulties.

Guidelines: (1) Help the couple to explore and restructure their attitudes toward sexual expression in line with their current goals and expectations for their relationship. (2) Discuss techniques to increase physical attractiveness and sexual responsiveness. (3) Encourage partners to communicate to each other their needs, including what is most pleasurable. (4) Suggest specific remedies for such common problems as anxiety and fatigue during intercourse, and introduce some alternate pleasuring methods to maintain intimacy. (5) Include the partner in sexual counseling and reassure him or her that physical exertion during intercourse is not harmful to the patient.

IT — Providing Intensive Therapy

Objective: Make appropriate referrals for sexual therapy when the patient is not responding to counseling or when the problems are related to a poor marriage.

Guidelines: (1) Provide for follow-up visits to evaluate response to sexual counseling. (2) Recognize limitations and refer to a competent sex therapist.

Note. Reprinted with permission from ''Sexual Counseling for the Chronic Obstructive Pulmonary Disease Patient'' by H.M. Kravetz, 1982, *Clinical Challenges in Cardiopulmonary Medicine,* **4,** pp. 1-6. Copyright 1982 by H.M. Kravetz.

are methods of evaluating compliance to determine therapeutic levels of drugs as seen in Table 3.4. Specific areas of training listed here should be covered regularly to insure compliance.

- Proper use of aerosolized medications[20,21]
- Medication use (see Table 3.4)
- Medication changes during an acute exacerbation
- Other areas of medications based upon the ongoing patient assessment

Respiratory Modalities

Depending on the patient's disease state, various respiratory modalities may be utilized to aid the patient in breathing. Additionally, individual patients may benefit from training programs covering such topics as nicotine dependency, environmental pollutants, and occupa-

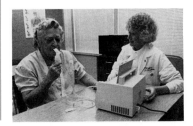

Table 3.4   Therapeutic Responses as Related to Blood Levels of Theophylline

Response	Blood level of theophylline
No effect	< 5 μg/ml
Suboptimal therapeutic level	5-9 μg/ml
Optimal therapeutic range	10-20 μg/ml
Anxiety may appear	> 15 μg/ml
GI toxicity likely	> 15 μg/ml
Usual toxic level	> 20 μg/ml
Arrhythmias likely to occur	> 30 μg/ml
Convulsions may occur	> 40 μg/ml

Note. Reprinted with permission from ''Pharmacology and the Respiratory Patient'' by A.R. Yee, G.L. Connors, and D.B. Cress. In *Pulmonary Rehabilitation: Guidelines to Success* (p. 129) by J.E. Hodgkin, E.G. Zorn, and G.L. Connors (Eds.). Copyright 1984 by J.E. Hodgkin.

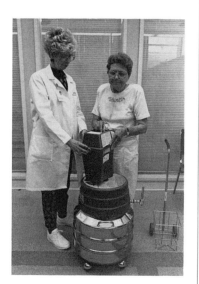

tional irritants. These areas are critical to optimizing the patient's ADL. Areas listed here should be addressed on an individual basis from information gathered during the initial assessment and reassessments.

- Nicotine dependency intervention[22,23]
- Secondhand smoke
- Environmental and occupational irritants
- Oxygen as a drug[24-26]
- Oxygen-conserving devices[27-29]
- Use, care, and cleaning of home respiratory equipment
- Suctioning in the home
- Ventilator management in the home[30,31]
- Sleep hygiene (apnea, oxygen desaturation, etc.)
- Home care
- Other areas of respiratory modalities based upon the ongoing patient assessment

Psychosocial Interventions

Chapter 5 covers in detail the area of psychosocial issues in pulmonary disease. Some patients will cope better than others with the emotional results that a chronic lung disease will produce. All pulmonary rehabilitation programs should address these issues on a regular basis during program sessions. The initial assessment should address the areas listed here, and the staff should intervene where appropriate on an individual basis.

- Coping with lung disease[32]
- Stress management techniques
- Support system and dependency issues
- Anger management
- Depression

- Self-efficacy for rehabilitation-related behaviors
- Other areas of psychosocial intervention based upon the ongoing patient assessment

Other areas of concern that may affect the patient's ability to benefit from rehabilitation include age, mental capacity, language, reading ability, and side effects of medications.[33] (See Table 3.4 on the use of medications.) Use of the health belief model and multidimensional health locus of control may aid the professional in better understanding the patient's concepts about his or her disease.[34] A list of the training resource material available to pulmonary rehabilitation programs is found in Appendix D.

The physical environment for patient training should be appropriate to the needs of pulmonary patients. Factors to be considered include proximity to parking, handicapped access, adequate space, ventilation and air conditioning, and bathroom access. The type of audiovisual equipment used will depend upon the training resource materials chosen and the program budget. A patient manual for use during and after the program is a helpful and important training tool. The design will vary with each program, but one cannot overemphasize the value of a simple, nontechnical presentation of the training material.[35,36] A patient training manual is a resource that the patient may utilize while participating in the program and after the program is completed. Included in this manual may be material relevant to the training program such as self-assessment tools, bronchial hygiene, activities of daily living, medications, respiratory modalities, and nutrition components inherent in dealing with chronic pulmonary disease. Appendix D presents a guide to the training resource material available to pulmonary rehabilitation programs. Every method of educational reinforcement that is available should be utilized in creating opportunities for better learning and understanding. Outcomes are facilitated by inputs and practice; this is what patient training is all about. (See chapter 7 for a discussion of facilities.)

The facility should ensure close proximity to parking and bathrooms, easy access for people with disabilities, sufficient space for training and exercise, and adequate ventilation.

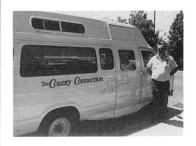

Conclusion

An effective pulmonary rehabilitation program helps the patient and significant others to develop a working knowledge of the patient's disease process and an appropriate, effective treatment program of self-care with symptom management. Team members develop an individualized rehabilitation program for each patient based on patient goals, incorporating the training sessions, exercise activities, and psychosocial interventions necessary for successful rehabilitation.

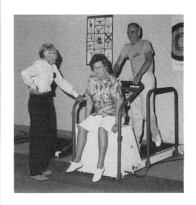

References

1. Hopp JW, Maddox ES. Education of patients and their families. In: Hodgkin JE, Zorn EG, Connors GL, eds. *Pulmonary Rehabilitation: Guidelines to Success*. Boston, Mass: Butterworth; 1984;5:45-65.
2. Bandura A. Self-efficacy: toward a unifying theory of behavioral change. *Psych Rev*. 1977;84:191-215.

3. Neish CM, Hopp JW. The role of education in pulmonary rehabilitation. *J Cardiop Rehab.* 1988;8(11):439-441.

4. Gilmartin ME. Patient and family education. *Clin Chest Med.* 1986;7(4):619-627.

5. Mast ME, VanAtta MJ. Applying adult learning principles in instructional module design. *Nurse Educator.* January/February 1986;11(1)35.

6. Knowles M. The adult learner: a neglected species. Houston, TX: Gulf Publishing Co, 1973;45-49.

7. Morris K, Russo A. *P.A.T.H. Positive Attitudes Toward Health: A Handbook on Pulmonary Rehabilitation.* Daly City, CA: Seton Medical Center; 1984:7.

8. Tiep B, Burns M, Kao D, Madison R, Herrera J. Pursed lip breathing training using ear oximetry. *Chest.* August 1986:5-29.

9. Faling LJ. Chest physical therapy. In: Burton GG, Hodgkin JE, Ward JJ, eds. *Respiratory Care: A Guide to Clinical Practice.* 3rd ed. Philadelphia, PA: JB Lippincott; 1991.

10. Hilling L, Bakow E, Fink J, Kelly C, Sobash D, Southorn P. AARC guidelines: postural drainage therapy. *Respiratory Care.* 1991;36(12):1418-1426.

11. Sutton PP, Parker RA, Webber BA, et al. Assessment of the forced expiration technique, postural drainage and directed coughing in chest physiotherapy. *Eur J Respir Dis.* 1983;64:62-68.

12. Bateman JRM, Newman SP, Daunt KM, et al. Is cough as effective as chest physiotherapy in the removal of excessive trancheobronchial secretions. *Thorax.* 1981;36:683-687.

13. Ragbeh M, Griffith H. The contribution of leisure participation and leisure satisfaction to life satisfaction of older persons. *Leisure Satisfaction Res.* 1982;4(14):295-306.

14. Tiep BL. *Portable Oxygen Therapy: Including Oxygen-Conserving Methodology.* New York, NY: Future Publishing Co; 1991.

15. Burns M. Social and recreational support of the pulmonary patient. In: Hodgkin JE, Connors GL, Bell CW, eds. *Pulmonary Rehabilitation: Guidelines to Success.* 2nd ed. Philadelphia, PA: JB Lippincott; 1992.

16. Kanner RE. Evaluation of impairment for disability determination. In: Hodgkin JE, Connors GL, Bell CW, eds. *Pulmonary Rehabilitation: Guidelines to Success.* 2nd ed. Philadelphia, PA: JB Lippincott; 1992.

17. Theodore AC, Beer DJ. Pharmacotherapy of chronic obstructive pulmonary disease. In: Make BJ, guest ed. *Pulmonary Rehabilitation. Clinics in Chest Med.* 7(4). Philadelphia, PA: WB Saunders; December 1986:657-672.

18. Ziment I. Drugs used in respiratory therapy. In: Burton GG, Hodgkin JE, Ward JJ, eds. *Respiratory Care: A Guide to Clinical Practice.* 3rd ed. Philadelphia, PA: JB Lippincott; 1991:411-448.

19. Jenne J. Pharmacology and use of respiratory medications in obstructive airway diseases. In: Hodgkin JE, Connors GL, Bell CW, eds. *Pulmonary Rehabilitation: Guidelines to Success.* 2nd ed. Philadelphia, PA: JB Lippincott; 1992.

20. Kacmarek RM, Vaz Fragoso CA. Aerosol therapy. In: Hodgkin JE, Connors GL, Bell CW, eds. *Pulmonary Rehabilitation: Guidelines to Success.* 2nd ed. Philadelphia, PA: JB Lippincott; 1992.

21. Consensus conference on aerosol delivery. Special issue, *Resp Care*. 1991;36(9):913-1044.

22. US Dept of Health and Human Services. The nicotine dependency program. NIH Pub #89.2961:1989; October: Part 1, 2 and 3.

23. Nett LM. *Smoking Cessation Resource List*. AARC publications; 1991:1-19.

24. Nocturnal oxygen therapy trial group. Continuous or nocturnal oxygen therapy in hypoxemic chronic obstructive lung disease: a clinical trial. *Ann Intern Med*. 1980;93:391-398.

25. Tiep BL. Long-term home oxygen therapy. In: Hodgkin JE, guest ed. *Chronic Obstructive Pulmonary Disease. Clin Chest Med*. 11(3):505-521. Philadelphia, PA: WB Saunders; September 1990.

26. Ryerson EG, Block AJ. Oxygen as a drug: clinical properties, benefits, modes and hazards of administration. In: Burton GG, Hodgkin JE, Ward JJ, eds. *Respiratory Care: A Guide to Clinical Practice*. 3rd ed. Philadelphia, PA: JB Lippincott; 1991:319-340.

27. Tiep BL, Lewis ML. Oxygen conservation and oxygen-conserving devices in chronic lung disease: a review. *Chest*. 1987;92:263-272.

28. Heimlich HJ, Carr GC. Transtracheal catheter technique for pulmonary rehabilitation. *Ann Otol Rhinol Laryngol*. 1985;94:502-504.

29. Christopher KL, Spofford BT, Brannin PK, Petty TL. Transtracheal oxygen therapy for refractory hypoxemia. *JAMA*. 1986;256:494-497.

30. Make BJ, Gilmartin ME. Care of ventilator-assisted individuals in the home and alternative community sites. In: Burton GG, Hodgkin JE, Ward JJ, eds. *Respiratory Care: A Guide to Clinical Practice*. 3rd ed. Philadelphia, PA: JB Lippincott; 1991.

31. Make B, Gilmartin M, Brody JS, et al. Rehabilitation of ventilator-dependent subjects with lung disease: the concept and initial experience. *Chest*. 1984;86:358-365.

32. Krop AD, Block AJ, Cohen E. Neuropsychiatric effects of continuous oxygen therapy in chronic obstructive pulmonary disease. *Chest*. 1973;64:317-322.

33. Eaton ML, Holloway RL. Patient comprehension of written drug information. *Am Hosp Pharm*. 1980;37:240-243.

34. Hopp JW, Gerken CM. Making an educational diagnosis to improve patient education. *Resp Care*. 1983;28(11):1456-1461.

35. Bailey WC, Manzella BA. Asthma workbook airs first for adults. *Profiles in Healthcare Marketing*. July 1991:80-83.

36. Lung disease care and education staff. *COPD Resource Guide*. New York, NY: American Lung Assoc; 1991:1-56.

Chapter 4

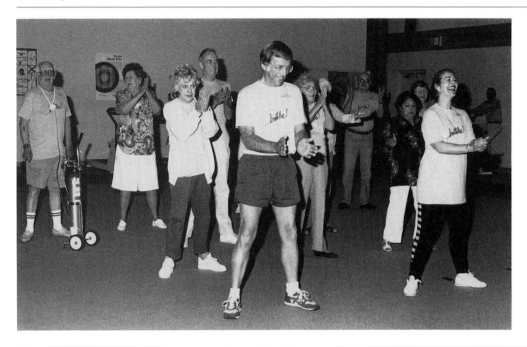

Exercise Testing and Training

Exercise is an important component of pulmonary rehabilitation programs. Each program should have appropriate facilities for testing and training patients. Exercise testing may be used to evaluate patients' exercise tolerance for training, to detect exercise hypoxemia, to assess the need for supplemental oxygen during training, and to evaluate cardiac function.[1,2] The benefits of exercise training for improving patients' functional capacity and activities of daily living have been well established (see Appendixes A and C).[3,4] Facilities and equipment will vary, depending upon resources as well as patient and program interests and needs.

Exercise testing and training are essential components of the pulmonary rehabilitation program.

Exercise Testing

A variety of exercise testing procedures and protocols have been used in evaluating patients for pulmonary rehabilitation programs. Methods range from simple, noninvasive procedures to complex, technically sophisticated, invasive procedures capable of measuring many variables. No single protocol has been clearly established as most appropriate for all patients and programs. Selection and design of an appropriate test depends upon individual patient goals, program objectives, questions identified in the initial patient evaluation, the exercise training program, available laboratory expertise, and cost.[2,5-7]

Equipment and Personnel Requirements

The requirements for exercise testing are these:

Minimal requirements

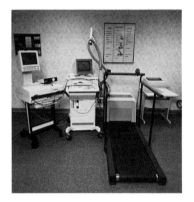

- A calibrated cycle ergometer or motorized treadmill (a measured walking distance may be used if no ergometer or treadmill is available). A step test, which is very simple and practical, may also be used.
- Manual blood pressure measurement equipment
- Cutaneous oximeter
- Oxygen source
- Access to a laboratory for arterial blood gas analysis
- Emergency plan and supplies (refer to hospital/facility policy)
- Test-site personnel trained in basic life-support techniques

Additional requirements

- EKG monitoring during exercise
- Defibrillator and crash cart
- Equipment for expired gas analysis to measure $\dot{V}O_2$, $\dot{V}CO_2$, minute ventilation, and derived variables (see Table 4.1)
- ACLS certification for test-site personnel

Table 4.1 Exercise Response Interpretation

Measurement	Deconditioning	Cardiac	COPD	Fibrosis	Pulmonary-vascular
$\dot{V}O_2$max	Low	Low	Low	Low	Low
HR/workload	High	High			High
MVV$-\dot{V}_E$max	High	High	Low	Low	
O_2sat			Low	Low	Extra Low
O_2 pulse		Low			Low
V_D/V_T			High	High	Extra High

Note. Reprinted with permission from "Pulmonary Function Tests" by P.L. Enright and J.E. Hodgkin. In *Respiratory Care: A Guide to Clinical Practice* (3rd ed.) (p. 175) by G.G. Burton, J.E. Hodgkin, and J.J. Ward (Eds.). Copyright 1991 by J.B. Lippincott.

Indications for Exercise Testing

Compared to exercise testing for healthy persons or cardiac patients, exercise testing in the diagnostic evaluation of pulmonary patients is at an early stage of development. Much more is known about what variables can be measured than about the indications for testing and the use and interpretation of test results for these patients. The following are some general guidelines about how exercise testing may be used in evaluating patients for pulmonary rehabilitation.

Measure Exercise Tolerance

Patients with chronic lung disease develop progressive dyspnea on exertion, which is a primary reason for their limited exercise tolerance. Dyspnea is a complex, subjective symptom of breathlessness at a level of exertion that the patient feels is abnormal.[8]

A schematic representation of the important role of reduced lung function in limiting exercise tolerance in pulmonary patients is depicted in Figure 4.1. Obstructive or restrictive lung disease leads to a reduction in forced expiratory volume in the first second (FEV_1), the lung function parameter most closely correlated with physical work capacity. This results in a decreased resting maximal voluntary ventilation (MVV approximated by $35 \times FEV_1$). The MVV is used to approximate the maximal ventilation ($\dot{V}_E max$) that can be reached during exercise. In turn, the reduced exercise $\dot{V}_E max$ limits oxygen transport ($\dot{V}O_2 max$). However, lung function alone cannot be used to predict exercise tolerance precisely because of the complex determinants of dyspnea. Therefore, it is necessary to exercise the pulmonary patient to a symptom-limited maximum in order to determine exercise tolerance.

It is necessary to exercise the pulmonary patient to a symptom-limited maximum in order to determine exercise tolerance.

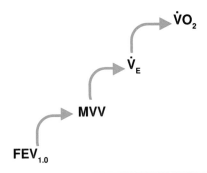

Figure 4.1 Schematic representation of the role of reduced lung function in limiting exercise tolerance in pulmonary patients. Lung disease leads to a reduction in $FEV_{1.0}$. This results in a decrease in the resting maximal voluntary ventilation (MVV = $35 \times FEV_{1.0}$) that approximates the maximal ventilatory reserve during exercise ($V_E max$). The reduction in $V_E max$ produces a ventilatory limitation to maximal oxygen transport ($\dot{V}O_2 max$) and exercise tolerance.

Note. Reprinted with permission from "The Role of Exercise Testing in Pulmonary Diagnosis" by A.L. Ries, 1987, *Clinics in Chest Medicine*, 8:81-89. Copyright 1987 by W.B. Saunders.

Out of a laboratory setting, exercise tolerance can be evaluated with a simple test such as a timed distance walk (e.g., a 6- or 12-minute walk).[9] In the exercise laboratory, more precise quantification of exercise performance can be made. The minimum measurements needed are work rate, heart rate, blood pressure, and preferably $\dot{V}_E$, so that the level of exercise ventilation can be related to resting pulmonary function. It is also helpful to have the patient rate the level of perceived breathlessness and muscle fatigue.[10] The additional option of expired gas analysis allows for $\dot{V}O_2$ measurement, the most accurate measure of metabolic work, and for noninvasive determination of the anaero-

Exercise testing measurements may include work rate, clinical signs and symptoms, electrocardiogram, ventilation, expired gas, and arterial blood gases.

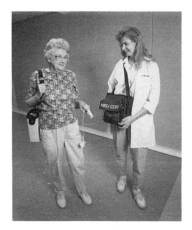

bic threshold, an important parameter of physical and cardiovascular fitness and an indicator of good patient effort. Many pulmonary patients whose exercise tolerance is limited by reduced ventilatory capacity do not, however, reach an anaerobic threshold.

Measurements of maximal exercise tolerance are helpful in planning exercise training programs and may be useful for assessing and following the functional impact of disease on a patient's physical work capacity.

Assess Exercise Limitation

In most patients being evaluated, the cause of dyspnea will be clear after the initial evaluation, including a review of the history and physical examination and screening laboratory data, including a chest radiograph, ABG, electrocardiogram, and pulmonary function tests. However, in some patients, the cause of dyspnea on exertion may still be unclear. In such situations, it may be useful to perform an incremental, maximal, symptom-limited exercise test to assess whether the patient has reduced exercise tolerance due to dyspnea and whether a cause for the dyspnea can be determined (e.g., ventilatory, cardiac, or other limitation to maximum exercise). Patients whose $\dot{V}_E$max approaches their resting MVV are considered to be ventilatory-limited. Patients with cardiac limitation will reach their predicted maximum heart rate (HRmax = $210 - [-0.65 \times$ age]; SD $\pm$ 10 beats/minute). Patients may also show other responses, giving clues to their exertional dyspnea (e.g., irregular breathing pattern or hyperventilation, suggesting a psychological cause of dyspnea).

In testing patients for unexplained dyspnea, it is preferable to perform both expired and arterial blood gas analyses. Measuring $\dot{V}O_2$max accurately quantifies maximum exercise tolerance. However, because many patients will not reach a true plateau in $\dot{V}O_2$ at maximum work rates, determination of anaerobic threshold may be helpful in assessing both cardiac and physical fitness and patient effort. Blood gas analysis is important in detecting significant exercise-induced hypoxemia as a factor contributing to dyspnea.

Assessing Blood Gas Changes

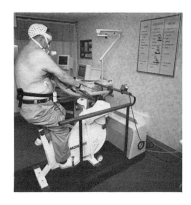

In patients with lung disease, blood gas measurements during exercise may be significantly different from those obtained at rest. Patients with interstitial lung disease typically develop widening of the alveolar-arterial oxygen gradient with exercise. This change has been proposed as a sensitive test to detect disease at an early stage.[11] In patients with obstructive lung disease, PaO_2 may change in an unpredictable manner during exercise. Some patients will develop significant exercise-induced hypoxemia, whereas in others the PaO_2 may not change or may even increase.[12] Unfortunately, there are no clinical features or resting measurements of pulmonary function or gas exchange that can predict the exercise response reliably. Therefore, it is necessary to measure blood gases during exercise to detect exercise-induced hypoxemia and to assess whether hypoxemia is contributing to the patient's complaint of exertional dyspnea. Such testing is also used for assessing a patient's response to supplemental oxygen in order to provide an accurate prescription for oxygen therapy at rest or with exercise (i.e., daily activities for many patients).

Because of the rapid changes in PaO_2 immediately after exercise, it is necessary to measure blood gases during exercise.[13] PaO_2 measured even 20 to 30 seconds after exercise may be significantly different from that obtained during exercise. An indwelling arterial catheter is generally required to obtain multiple blood samples rapidly for such tests. Newer, noninvasive techniques such as cutaneous oximetry from measuring arterial oxygen saturation are useful for continuous monitoring, but have a limited absolute accuracy (95% confidence limits $\pm$ 3% to 5% saturation).[14]

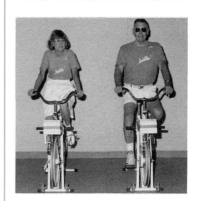

Exercise-Induced Bronchospasm

Patients with airway hyperreactivity (e.g., asthmatics) commonly develop worsening expiratory flow rates with an exercise challenge (exercise-induced bronchospasm). This may occur in patients with or without recognized lung disease. Therefore, in exercising pulmonary patients, it is important to have a high index of suspicion for worsening symptoms of breathlessness during exercise related to exercise-induced changes in lung function. If such a condition is suspected, monitoring lung function (e.g., spirometry) before and after exercise may help to detect it.[15]

Type of Exercise

In general, exercise performance is relatively specific to activities and the muscles used. Therefore, exercise tests should be designed to correspond to the planned exercise training program. For most clinical purposes, testing uses exercise of the large muscles of the trunk and lower extremities to produce high levels of physiological stress and because training programs typically involve lower extremity exercise (e.g., walking, cycling).

Simple tests such as the Master's step test or the timed walking distance (e.g., 6- or 12-minute walk) do not require sophisticated equipment and can be used to assess a patient's exercise tolerance and limiting symptoms. If available, a calibrated cycle ergometer or motorized treadmill provides more precise quantification of mechanical work load and keeps the patient in one place to allow for more complex measurements when needed.

With a cycle ergometer mechanically braked by a strap, work rate (power) depends on pedaling frequency, which must be controlled. An electrically braked cycle ergometer is less dependent on pedaling rate, although it is more expensive. For treadmills used in testing or training disabled pulmonary patients, slow speeds are necessary. The minimum treadmill speed should be at least 1.0 mph and, preferably, less than 1.0 mph for the more disabled patients.

Laboratory Testing Protocols

In the laboratory setting, exercise testing protocols used for evaluating pulmonary patients typically include two general types: incremental and steady-state. For incremental tests, the work load is increased at a predetermined interval (e.g., 1 minute) to a maximum, symptom-limited level. Ideally, the subject should reach his or her maximum within 10 to 15 minutes. The size of the work increments depends on the patient: Smaller steps are used for more limited patients. On a cycle ergometer, work may be increased by 10 to 15 watts (60 to 90

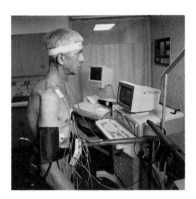

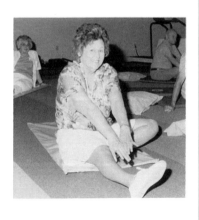

kpm/minute) each minute. On a treadmill, speed can be increased in 0.5 mph steps up to 3.0 mph; further work increments can be made by increasing elevation by 2%. These rapid, multiple-stage tests are most useful for assessing maximal exercise tolerance and for evaluating the pattern of physiological response to increasing work loads.

In steady-state tests (single- or multiple-stage), work load is maintained at a constant level for a predetermined period of time to allow the subject to reach steady state for the variables of interest. Healthy persons usually reach a steady state within 4 to 5 minutes; pulmonary patients may take longer. For rehabilitation program uses, such tests can be useful in assessing baseline levels for subsequent exercise training or determining the need for and prescribing supplemental oxygen therapy.

Measurements

The type of measurements made during exercise testing will depend upon the purpose and type of test. In any test it is important to quantify the work rate achieved. In addition, for testing pulmonary patients, other variables may be measured and/or monitored.

Work Rate

For simple exercise tests such as a timed-walk test, work rate will be measured by the maximum distance covered in a given time period (e.g., 6 or 12 minutes). In the laboratory, mechanical work may be measured in watts (kpm/minute) for a cycle ergometer or by speed and grade on a treadmill.

Clinical Signs and Symptoms

For all exercise tests of pulmonary patients, it is important to describe and characterize signs and symptoms that occur during (and limit) exercise. Although dyspnea (breathlessness) will limit exercise in many patients, other limiting symptoms (e.g., muscle fatigue) are also common. Appropriate interpretation of the test requires an assessment of the clinical symptoms. Therefore, patients should be asked specifically about shortness of breath, muscle fatigue, chest pain, or other symptoms and examined for signs of increased wheezing. Ratings of perceived symptoms (e.g., breathlessness, fatigue) can be used to characterize and quantify these clinical findings (by using the Perceived Symptom Scale in Figure 4.2).[10]

Electrocardiogram

For exercise testing in pulmonary patients, a single (modified V5) lead is typically used to measure heart rate and to monitor for arrhythmias or ischemic changes. Full 12-lead monitoring is not necessary for all pulmonary patients unless ischemic heart disease is suspected. Blood pressure should be measured at regular intervals.

Ventilation

Total expired (or inspired) ventilation can be measured to assess the ventilatory response to exercise. This may help to quantify the ventilatory reserve with exercise. For this measurement, a low-resistance, low-dead-space breathing valve connected to a mouthpiece is used to

0	Nothing at all
0.5	Very, very slight (just noticeable)
1	Very slight
2	Slight
3	Moderate
4	Somewhat severe
5	Severe
6	
7	Very severe
8	
9	Very, very severe (almost maximum)
10	Maximum

Figure 4.2 Perceived symptom scale used to rate symptoms of breathlessness and fatigue during exercise testing.

Note. Reprinted with permission from G.A. Borg, "Psychophysical Bases of Perceived Exertion," *Medicine and Science in Sports and Exercise*, Volume 14, pp. 377-387, 1982, © by the American College of Sports Medicine.

separate inspired from expired air. Expired gas can be collected in a Tissot spirometer or Douglas bag, or analyzed continuously by a flow-measuring device (e.g., a pneumotachograph). Inspired volume can also be measured by a dry gas meter. Respiratory rate and tidal volume (V_T) may also be monitored. The normal ventilatory response to exercise involves an increase in both respiratory rate and V_T to produce an increase in total ventilation.

The type of measurements made during exercise testing will depend on the purpose and type of test.

Expired Gas Analysis

Measurement of O_2 and CO_2 in the expired gas by calibrated gas analyzers allows calculation of oxygen uptake ($\dot{V}O_2$), carbon dioxide output ($\dot{V}CO_2$), and other derived variables such as ventilatory equivalents O_2 ($\dot{V}_E/\dot{V}O_2$) and CO_2 ($\dot{V}_E/\dot{V}CO_2$), respiratory exchange ratio (R = $\dot{V}CO_2/\dot{V}O_2$), and oxygen pulse ($\dot{V}O_2$/heart rate). Performing these measurements in response to an exercise challenge may help to better understand the response to exercise and limitations but are not necessary for all patients entering a rehabilitation program. $\dot{V}O_2$ is the best measurement of the metabolic requirement of work; $\dot{V}O_2$max is the standard measurement of exercise capacity. CO_2 is produced both as a by-product of aerobic metabolism and from bicarbonate buffering of lactic acid under anaerobic conditions. Analysis of the triphasic ventilatory response during a rapid incremental work test allows determination of the anaerobic threshold, the point at which significant anaerobic metabolism ensues. This is an important parameter reflecting physical and cardiac fitness, but it might not be reached by many patients with chronic lung disease.[16]

Arterial Blood Gases

In contrast to healthy persons who maintain normal arterial levels of oxygen (PaO_2) and carbon dioxide ($PaCO_2$) during exercise, pulmonary patients may develop significant changes. Because of rapid changes in PaO_2 immediately after exercise, arterial blood needs to be sampled during exercise.[13] An indwelling catheter is needed to collect multiple samples rapidly. This significantly increases the complexity, patient discomfort, and cost of testing. Newer, noninvasive methods for assessing arterial oxygenation, such as cutaneous oximeters, are promising for continuous monitoring within the limitations of absolute accuracy (95% confidence limits $\pm$ 3% to 5% for arterial oxygen saturation [SaO_2]).[14] However, relying solely on oximetry in assessing a pulmonary patient's need for supplemental oxygen therapy may provide misleading information in a significant proportion of patients.[17]

The alveolar-arterial oxygen gradient $P(A - a)O_2$ is the best parameter for assessing pulmonary oxygenation; alveolar PO_2 (PAO_2) is calculated most accurately with simultaneous measurements of $PaCO_2$ and respiratory exchange ratio (R), which requires expired gas analysis. Measurement of $PACO_2$ may be used to assess the adequacy of the ventilatory response to exercise. Also, in combination with simultaneous measurement of expired CO_2 concentration, dead-space (wasted) ventilation ($\dot{V}_D$) and V_D/V_T ratio can be calculated (normal V_D/V_T, 30% to 35% at rest, decreasing to less than 30% with exercise).

Exercise Training

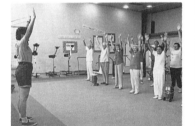

Developing and implementing a home exercise program is an important goal for all patients in pulmonary rehabilitation (see Appendix A, pp. 88-93).[18] In addition to improving physical work tolerance, it provides patients with opportunities to practice breathing techniques, and to control symptoms of breathlessness. Breathing control and pursed-lip breathing should be addressed before the patient begins an exercise program. This component is often neglected. The patient cannot achieve maximum exercise potential if she or he cannot optimally control breathing. The home exercise program should be pleasant and fulfilling, so that the patient looks forward to it rather than dreads it. Exercise may also be used as a social experience (e.g., to exercise with a friend, attend an exercise maintenance group, or walk in a mall). Home exercise should be an enjoyable and welcome change to a previously sedentary lifestyle.

There is considerable controversy about the best methods of prescribing exercise for patients with chronic pulmonary disease. A variety of training methods have been used successfully in pulmonary rehabilitation. Typically, programs tend to emphasize improving endurance through progressive training to symptom limits. It is important to start severely disabled patients at relatively low exercise levels and increase them as tolerated in small increments to build the patient's confidence and endurance. Because of the potential for exercise-associated hypoxemia in many patients, the information from the exercise test should be used to determine the need for supplemental oxygen with exercise. In such patients, program staff should review options for oxygen therapy, instruct the patient in its proper use, and reevaluate oxygen need and prescription as the patient progresses through the program.

To set up an exercise program, four components should be determined:

- Duration
- Frequency
- Intensity
- Mode[19]

The staff should determine duration, frequency, intensity, and mode of a patient's exercise program.

The duration of an endurance exercise session is typically set at a goal of 20 to 30 minutes of continuous activity plus warm-up and cool-down periods, including stretching. Many patients start training for shorter time periods and progress as tolerated. This allows them to gain confidence, improve their self-efficacy, and work toward their goals.

Exercise frequency should be a minimum of 3 days per week, for a training effect to be reached and maintained. During exacerbations, patients should be instructed to reduce their exercise program as tolerated until they recover.

Pulmonary rehabilitation programs have used different approaches to intensity for exercise training. Some use a target heart rate (THR). Karvonen's formula using 0.6 as the intensity factor has been reported to provide an initial THR that is acceptable for many COPD patients[20]:

$$\text{Target HR} = [0.6 \times (\text{Peak HR} - \text{Resting HR})] + \text{Resting HR}$$

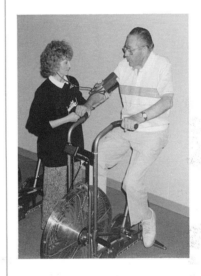

The advantage of Karvonen's formula for determining target heart rate is that it takes into consideration both peak and resting heart rates. Because many pulmonary patients have higher resting heart rates, using a fixed percentage of peak heart rate (e.g., 0.7 × Peak HR) may calculate a target heart rate lower than the patient's resting heart rate. Alternative approaches for exercise intensity have used symptom-limited targets (e.g., a target level of perceived breathlessness). It has been shown that many of the more severe ventilatory-limited patients can reach levels during training that approach 100% of maximum exercise tolerance and that COPD patients who exercise at an intensity above their anaerobic threshold achieve more improvement in exercise capacity than those training at a lower level.[16,21]

During exercise training sessions, minimum routine patient monitoring should consist of heart rate and dyspnea level. If indicated, oximetry and blood pressure should be monitored.

A variety of exercise training modalities have been used successfully in pulmonary rehabilitation. The most common is walking, but other aerobic-type exercises are treadmill, cycling, stationary bicycle, step exercise, rowing, water exercises, swimming, and modified aerobic dance. There is some evidence that upper extremity exercises, such as arm cycling, as well as simple exercises of arm lifts with and without weights, may be particularly useful for pulmonary patients.[22] Many studies of ventilatory muscle training have demonstrated improvements in ventilatory muscle performance, but there is no definite evidence that adding respiratory muscle training to a pulmonary rehabilitation program that includes an aerobic exercise training program improves functional activity, quality of life, survival, or reduces

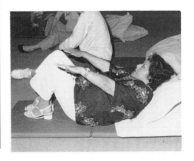

morbidity.[23] In addition, some programs utilize resistive training devices to improve strength in these patients. Whichever type of exercise program is used for an individual patient, it is important to document the patient's progress throughout the rehabilitation program.

Emergency Procedures

It is important to have appropriate emergency plans and supplies in the exercise training facilities. All staff should be familiar with the hospital/facility procedures for cardiopulmonary resuscitation (CPR). Minimum cardiopulmonary general emergency equipment should include an oxygen source and delivery apparatus, resuscitation bag and mask, first aid supplies, and bronchodilator medications. In addition, personnel who work with pulmonary patients should be familiar with emergency procedures for these patients. In the acutely dyspneic patient, the following may be recommended:

1. Have the patient stop activity and assume a comfortable breathing position.
2. Encourage the patient to use pursed-lip breathing and relaxation techniques.
3. Use bronchodilator medication, if indicated.
4. Monitor oxygen saturation, if equipment is available.

Conclusion

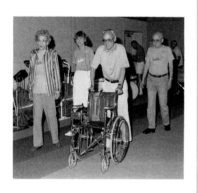

The importance of an exercise training program cannot be overemphasized. But before a safe program can be outlined, a thorough assessment needs to be done to detect exercise hypoxemia, to assess the need for supplemental oxygen during training, and to evaluate cardiac function. The well-documented benefits of exercise training include increased tolerance for dyspnea, improved appetite, increased physical capability, and an improved quality of life. Exercise is one of the essential components of a comprehensive pulmonary rehabilitation program.

References

1. Ries AL. The role of exercise testing in pulmonary diagnosis. *Clinics in Chest Med*. 1987;8:81-89.
2. Belman MJ, Wasserman K. Exercise testing and training in patients with chronic obstructive pulmonary disease. *Basics of RD*. 1981;10:1-6.
3. Belman MJ. Exercise in chronic obstructive pulmonary disease. In: Make BJ, ed. *Pulmonary Rehabilitation. Clinics in Chest Med*. 1986;7:585-597.
4. Hughes RL, Davison R. Limitations of exercise reconditioning in COLD. *Chest*. 1983;83:241-249.
5. Jones NL. *Clinical Exercise Testing*. 3rd ed. Philadelphia, PA: WB Saunders, 1988.

6. Wasserman K, Hansen JE, Sue DY, Whipp BJ. *Principles of Exercise Testing and Interpretation*. Philadelphia, PA: Lea & Febiger; 1987.

7. Spiro SG. Exercise testing in clinical medicine. *Br J Dis Chest*. 1977;71:145-172.

8. Mahler DA. *Dyspnea*. Mount Kisco, NY: Futura Publishing Co, 1990.

9. McGavin CR, Gupta SP, McHardy GJR. Twelve-minute walking test for assessing disability in chronic bronchitis. *Br Med J*. 1976;1:822-823.

10. Borg GAV. Psychophysical bases of perceived exertion. *Med Sci Sports Exer*. 1982;14:377-381.

11. Keogh BA, Lakatos E, Price D, Crystal RG. Importance of the lower respiratory tract in oxygen transfer: exercise testing in patients with interstitial and destructive lung disease. *Am Rev Respir Dis*. 1984;129:S76-S80.

12. Ries AL, Farrow JT, Clausen JL. Pulmonary function tests cannot predict exercise-induced hypoxemia in chronic obstructive pulmonary disease. *Chest*. 1988;93:454-459.

13. Ries AL, Fedullo PF, Clausen JL. Rapid changes in arterial blood gas levels after exercise in pulmonary patients. *Chest*. 1983;83:454-456.

14. Ries AL, Farrow JT, Clausen JL. Accuracy of two ear oximeters at rest and during exercise in pulmonary patients. *Am Rev Respir Dis*. 1985;132:685-689.

15. Anderson SD. Exercise-induced asthma: the state of the art. *Chest*. 1985;87:191S-195S.

16. Punzal PA, Ries AL, Kaplan RM, Prewitt LP. Maximum intensity exercise training in patients with chronic obstructive pulmonary disease. *Chest*. 1991;100:618-623.

17. Carlin BW, Clausen JL, Ries AL. The use of cutaneous oximetry in the prescription of long-term oxygen therapy. *Chest*. 1988;94:239-241.

18. Hodgkin JE. Exercise testing and training. In: Hodgkin JE, Petty TL, eds. *Chronic Obstructive Pulmonary Disease: Current Concepts*. Philadelphia, PA: WB Saunders, 1987;120.

19. Bell CW. Pulmonary rehabilitation and exercise. In: Wilson PK, Bell CW, Norton AC, eds. *Rehabilitation of the Heart and Lungs*. Fullterton, Calif: Beckman Instruments; 1980:54.

20. Hodgkin JE, Litzau KL. Exercise training target heart rates in chronic obstructive pulmonary disease. *Chest*. 1988;94:305.

21. Litzau KL, Hodgkin JE, Connors GL, Bickford CE. Determination of exercise training intensity in pulmonary patients. Abstract. *J Cardiop Rehab*. 1988;8:403.

22. Ellis B, Ries AL. Upper extremity exercise training in pulmonary rehabilitation. *J Cardiop Rehab*. 1991;11:227-231.

23. Pardy RL, Rochester DF. Respiratory muscle training. *Sem Respir Mod*. 1992;13:53-62.

Chapter 5

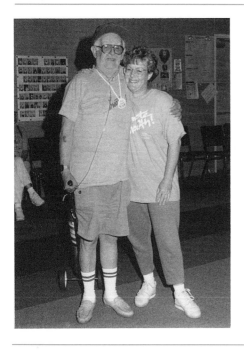

Psychosocial Components of a Comprehensive Program

Psychosocial problems play an important role in the symptomatology and problems of patients with chronic pulmonary diseases.[1-5] In the early stages of disease, patients and significant others are often unaware of, or deny the existence and seriousness of, their disease. Unlike the effects of other well-known diseases, the disabling effects and progression of chronic pulmonary diseases are not well known to the public. In the later stages of disease, patients may develop a variety of psychosocial symptoms reflecting progressive feelings of hopelessness and inability to cope with a disease process they do not understand. Depression is common and can be identified through simple screening tools.[6,7] Patients may also develop fear and anxiety[5] (particularly associated with breathlessness), anger, frustration, hostility, panic, irritability, psychosomatic symptoms, sexual problems, and cognitive and neuropsychological dysfunction.[1,8]

Pulmonary patients may develop feelings of hopelessness and the inability to cope with their disease process.

Psychosocial Assessment

In planning an individualized rehabilitation program for each patient, it is essential to evaluate the patient's psychological and emotional state

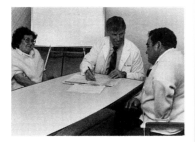

as well as his or her social support system. This evaluation may include a standardized questionnaire or information gathered in the interview with the patient and significant others. Examples of psychosocial measurements that may be considered due to their simplicity in administration, scoring, and interpretation are found in Table 5.1.[2] These tests are valid and reliable. Assessment areas generally include the following:

- Depression
- Anxiety
- Anger management
- Effectiveness of patient's rehabilitation-related behaviors
- Family support and dependency issues
- Perception of stress
- Coping styles
- General neuropsychological status
- Overall adaptation to illness
- Drug usage
- Compliance to medical regimens
- Impact of role change

Table 5.1 Psychosocial Measurements Useful in the Pulmonary Rehabilitation Patient Evaluation

Berle Index for Psychosocial Assets
Holmes and Rabe's Schedule of Recent Experience
Oar's Social Resource Scale
Self-Rating Depression Scale by Zung
Short Portable Mental Status Questionnaire
Rotter's Internal and External Locus of Control Scale
The Sickness Impact Profile
Health Attitude Test (Beck Depression Inventory)

Note. Adapted with permission from "Psychosocial Factors and Pulmonary Patients" by H.T. Kim, P.A. Knecht, D.E. Hiscox, and E.M. Glaser. In *Pulmonary Rehabilitation: Guidelines to Success* (pp. 216-218) by J.E. Hodgkin, E.G. Zorn, and G.L. Connors (Eds.). Copyright 1984 by J.E. Hodgkin.

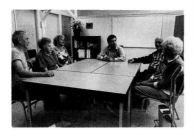

The patient often experiences both internal and external forces that affect the rehabilitative potential. Woolfolk[9] developed a multimodal model that looks at how psychosocial decisions are made, based upon the patient's internal dysfunctions and maladaptations to life situations. This profile—BASIC ID—stands for behavior, affect, sensory, imagery, cognition, interpersonal relationships, and drugs. A modification of this profile can be seen in Table 5.2.[2]

To look into the external forces that affect the patient's rehabilitation potential, the SELF model profile is useful.[2] SELF stands for support system, events, living conditions, and financial situations. See Table 5.3 for an example on the usage of the SELF profile.

Table 5.2 BASIC ID—Internal Modality Profile

	Modality	Problem	Proposed treatment
B	Behavior	Speech nonfluency	Behavior rehearsal
A	Affect	Mistrust and/or fear of spouse	Desensitization
S	Sensory	Muscular tension	Relaxation training
I	Imagery	Unrealistic scenes of retaliation	Self-hypnosis with success imagery
C	Cognition	Defeatist self-expression; irrational beliefs concerning physical illness	Modification of content of self-talk; rational disputation and bibliotherapy
I	Interpersonal	Lack of interpersonal sensitivity; control of spouse through passivity and withholding; reinforcement of passive role by spouse	Train in perception of nonverbal cues; train spouse to recognize and reinforce assertive behavior
D	Disease or reaction to drug	Shortness of breath; malnutrition	If necessary, discuss with physician

Note. Reprinted with permission from ''Psychosocial Factors and Pulmonary Patients'' by H.T. Kim, P.A. Knecht, D.E. Hiscox, and E.M. Glaser. In *Pulmonary Rehabilitation: Guidelines to Success* (p. 215) by J.E. Hodgkin, E.G. Zorn, and G.L. Connors (Eds.). Copyright 1984 by J.E. Hodgkin.

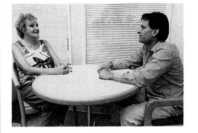

Table 5.3 SELF—External Modality Profile

	Modality	Problem	Proposed treatment
S	Support system	Lives with spouse, but spouse has hip fracture	Homemaker service arrangement
E	Events	Spouse's hip fracture; unseasonal flooding of home	Finding community resources for care and and assistance
L	Living conditions	Lives out of town where there is no public transportation; no transportation for medical appointments	Transportation arrangement; ''Meals-on-Wheels'' service
F	Financial status	Tight but manageable	Information on budget management agencies and public assistance programs

Note. Reprinted with permission from ''Psychosocial Factors and Pulmonary Patients'' by H.T. Kim, P.A. Knecht, D.E. Hiscox, and E.M. Glaser. In *Pulmonary Rehabilitation: Guidelines to Success* (p.216) by J.E. Hodgkin, E.G. Zorn, and G.L. Connors (Eds.). Copyright 1984 by J.E. Hodgkin.

Findings from the psychosocial screening should be integrated into the overall pulmonary rehabilitation plan with appropriate goals set for the treatment of specific psychosocial needs. Once the psychosocial assessment is completed, the treatment outlined can measure patient outcomes. The psychosocial interventions listed below may also be integrated throughout the pulmonary program, similar to what the patients are expected to do when they return home. For patients with more severe problems, referral to mental health professionals should be discussed with the patient's primary care physician.

Interventions

The purpose of psychosocial interventions in pulmonary rehabilitation is to help patients restore their self-esteem, learn adaptive coping skills (see Appendix A, pp. 86-88), and control or manage their symptoms. Interventions are based upon data gathered from the initial assessment. Knowledge of the patients' personal strengths, weaknesses, levels of performance, investment in their rehabilitation program, and the resources available to them will facilitate intervention design. Agle and Baum have shown that components of the pulmonary rehabilitation program lead to improved performance and psychosocial status. These components in particular are exercise, leading to a decrease in fear related to dyspnea; improvement in activities of daily living leading to greater independence; a sense of self-importance acquired from the rehabilitation team's attitudes; and the determination of realistic and achievable goals, which leads to improved self-esteem.[10] Consistent follow-up, review of status and achievement, and continued support received from group interaction are factors that lead to an increase in patient motivation.[10] The goal of the psychosocial intervention with each patient is to increase participation, confidence, and ego-strength. This can be achieved by enhancing the factors that lead to improved psychosocial status, as cited in Agle and Baum.

Many of the psychosocial concerns experienced by pulmonary patients may be addressed during other program activities by warm, caring, and supportive staff who are sensitive to the problems and needs of these patients. A regular support group may be helpful in addressing psychosocial needs of both patients and significant others. For certain patients, individual counseling may be appropriate and be provided either by a trained staff member or by referral to a mental health professional (after consultation with the primary care physician and/or the pulmonary rehabilitation medical director). Use of psychotropic medications (e.g., antidepressants) may be considered and recommended for some patients.[8]

Specific areas of concern for pulmonary patients include sexual dysfunction, inappropriate coping strategies, role reversal, social dependency, isolation, and economic hardship. Methods of stress management and relaxation therapy, including muscle tension relaxation or visualization, are also options to consider, based upon the individual patient's needs.

Although exercise has been found to reduce breathlessness, anxiety, and depression in the COPD patient[11-13] it should not be considered a panacea. A multimodal approach—from progressive muscle relaxa-

Psychosocial interventions help patients restore their self-esteem, learn adaptive coping skills, and control or manage their symptoms.

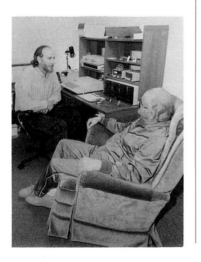

tion,[14] to biofeedback,[15] to other types of traditional psychotherapy[16,17]—may be necessary to meet the patient's individual needs.

Other areas that psychosocial interventions may address are counseling, facilitation of resources, and patient advocacy. Assisting the patient in the recognition and management of stressors may eliminate or assist in coping with areas that cause stress. Individual counseling, family therapy, group therapy, community support groups, outpatient home-care follow-up, vocational counseling, and psychiatric consultation are all potential treatment interventions.

Ethical Issues

Many of the patients in pulmonary rehabilitation programs have severe disease and limited life expectancy. Program staff must take an active role in helping all patients understand issues related to, and prepare for, death and dying. Staff should be able to provide, when appropriate, information and counseling on advanced directives, which may include resuscitation decisions, the living will, the durable power of attorney for health care, directives to physicians, and local resources for additional information and services.[18,19] For limiting the medical intervention given by paramedics in the home environment, other rules, forms, or laws may specifically apply. Check with the county medical society to verify resuscitation procedures in the home.

Conclusion

Utilization of the many assessment tools available to evaluate psychosocial function is essential in presenting a total pulmonary rehabilitation program. Psychological impairments have a direct and integrated influence on physical condition and response. The psychosocial evaluation and treatment should not be considered as a stand-alone component of the rehabilitation program, but should be integrated into all components of the program from the initial assessment through follow-up. Psychosocial intervention may include exercise, specific behavioral approaches, stress reduction, relaxation, counseling, and psychiatric evaluation. Success in pulmonary rehabilitation is achieved by using a comprehensive program, of which psychosocial intervention and well-being are a part.

Psychosocial impairments have a direct influence on physical condition and response.

References

1. Glaser EM, Dudley DL. Psychosocial rehabilitation and psychopharmacology. In: Hodgkin JE, Petty TL, eds. *Chronic Obstructive Pulmonary Disease: Current Concepts.* Philadelphia, PA: WB Saunders; 1987:128-153.
2. Kim HT, Knecht PA, Hiscox DE, Glaser EM. Psychosocial factors and pulmonary patients. In: Hodgkin JE, Zorn EG, Connors GL, eds. *Pulmonary Rehabilitation—Guidelines to Success.* Boston, Mass: Butterworth; 1984:207.

3. Ries AL. Position paper of the American Association of Cardiovascular and Pulmonary Rehabilitation. Scientific basis of pulmonary rehabilitation. *J Cardiop Rehab*. 1990;10:418-441.

4. Guyatt GH, Townsend M, Berman LB, Pugsley SD. Quality of life in patients with chronic airflow limitations. *Br J Dis Chest*. 1987;81:45.

5. Prigatano GP, Wright EC, Levin D. Quality of life and its predictors in patients with mild hypoxemia and chronic obstructive pulmonary disease. *Arch Intern Med*. 1984;144:1613-1619.

6. Agle DP, Baum GL. Psychological aspects of chronic obstructive pulmonary disease. *Med Clin of N Amer*. 1977;61:749-758.

7. McSweeny AJ, Grant I, Heaton RK, Adams KM, Timms RM. Life quality of patients with chronic obstructive pulmonary disease. *Arch of Int Med*. 1982;142:473-478.

8. Dudley DL, Glaser EM, Jorgenson BN, Logan DL. Psychosocial concomitants to rehabilitation in chronic obstructive pulmonary disease. *Chest*. 1980;77:677-684.

9. Woolfolk RL. The multimodal model as a framework for decision-making in psychotherapy. In: Lazarus AA, ed. *Multimodal Behavior Therapy*. New York, NY: Springer; 1976.

10. Agle DF, Baum GL, Chester EH, Wends M. Multidiscipline treatment of chronic pulmonary insufficiency. *Psychosom Med*. 1973;35(1):41-49.

11. McGavin CR, Gupta SP, Lloyd EL, McHardy JR. Physical rehabilitation of chronic bronchitis: results of a controlled trial of exercises in the home. *Thorax*. 1977;32:307.

12. Gayle RC, Spitler DL, Karper WB, Jaeger RM, Rice SN. Psychological changes in exercising COPD patients. *Int J Rehab Research*. 1988;11:335.

13. Emery CF, Leatherman NE, Burker EJ, MacIntyre NR. Psychological outcomes of a pulmonary rehabilitation program. *Chest*, in press.

14. Renfroe KL. Effect of progressive relaxation on dyspnea and state of anxiety in patients with chronic obstructive pulmonary disease. *Heart & Lung*. 1988;17:408.

15. Parker SR. Behavioral science aspects of COPD: current status and future directions. In: McSweeny AJ, Grant I, eds. *Chronic Obstructive Pulmonary Disease: A Behavioral Perspective*. New York, NY: Marcel Dekker Inc; 1988.

16. Greenberg GD, Ryan JJ, Bourlier PE. Psychological and neuropsychological aspects of COPD. *Psychosom*. 1985;26:29.

17. Lustig FM, Haas A, Castillo R. Clinical and rehabilitation regime in patients with chronic obstructive pulmonary disease. *Arch Phys Med Rehab*. 1972;53:315.

18. *Summary of California Law on Medical Decisionmaking*. California consortium on patient self determination, 1st ed. September 1991; 7-1—7-18.

19. Nett LM, Petty TL. Reconciliary ethical principles and new technology: a commentary on critical care medicine and mechanical ventilation. *Respir Care*. 1985;30:610-620.

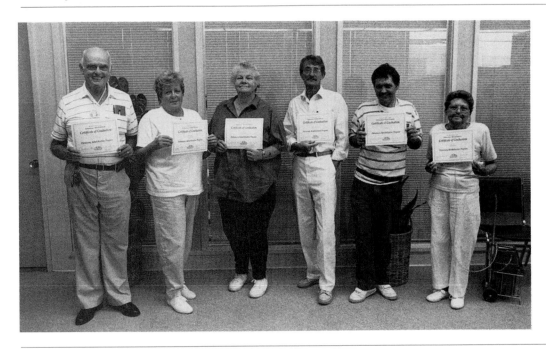

Chapter 6

Patient Outcomes, Program Follow-Up, and Continuous Quality Improvement

Comprehensive pulmonary rehabilitation can enhance both survival and outcomes for pulmonary rehabilitation patients.[1,2] Rehabilitation improves patients' quality of life, and the earlier it is started, the better the survival rate. Favorable outcomes are also seen in the elderly and patients with severe lung disease.[3]

Patient Outcomes and Program Follow-Up

In designing a pulmonary rehabilitation program, it is important to incorporate a plan for evaluating success in meeting program and patient goals. The specific components of this evaluation vary depending on the structure of the program. Formal research-based evaluation studies are not necessary, but information should be collected on an ongoing basis according to the specific program and patient goals. Areas that may be addressed are changes in exercise tolerance; onset,

Rehabilitation improves the patient's quality of life. The earlier it is started, the better the survival rate.

Patient progress should be evaluated on an ongoing basis.

55

frequency, and type of symptoms; and compliance with and adherence to medication regimens and the home program recommendations. See Table 6.1 for examples of types of information to be collected.[4-13]

To improve patient compliance and maintain long-term benefits, pulmonary rehabilitation programs have implemented various types of follow-up activities for their graduates. Maintenance exercise groups, outings, trips, newsletters, and phone calls are a few examples of follow-up activities. These have been shown to improve compliance with the home program plan. See Table 6.2 for further listing of follow-up options.

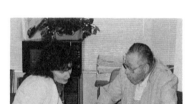

Table 6.1 Evaluating Patient Outcomes

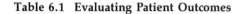

Changes in exercise tolerance
  Pre- and post-6- or 12-minute walk
  Pre- and postpulmonary exercise stress test
  Review of patient home exercise training logs
  Strength measurement
  Flexibility and posture
  Performance on specific training modalities (e.g., ventilatory muscle, upper extremity)

Changes in symptoms
  Dyspnea measurements comparison
  Frequency of cough, sputum production, or wheezing
  Weight gain or loss
  Psychological test instruments

Other changes
  Activities of Daily Living changes
  Postprogram follow-up questionnaires
  Pre/postprogram knowledge test
  Compliance improvement with pulmonary rehabilitation medical regimen
  Frequency and duration of respiratory exacerbations
  Frequency and duration of hospitalizations
  Frequency of emergency room visits
  Return to productive employment

Note. Reprinted with permission from "Organization and Management of a Pulmonary Rehabilitation Program" by L. Beytas and G.L. Connors. In *Pulmonary Rehabilitation: Guidelines to Success* (2nd ed.) by J.E. Hodgkin, G.L. Connors, and C.W. Bell (Eds.). Copyright 1992 by J. B. Lippincott.

Table 6.2 Follow-Up Options for Pulmonary Rehabilitation Programs

Regular physician visits
Maintenance exercise group
Program graduate group outings and trips
Program graduate group meetings

Referral to community groups (e.g., American Lung Association's "Better Breathers Clubs")

Phone follow-up by program staff

Newsletters

Postprogram questionnaires

Re-evaluation as indicated

Home-health referral

Home visits

National Pulmonary Rehabilitation Week (observed during the first week of spring)

Note. Reprinted with permission from "Organization and Management of a Pulmonary Rehabilitation Program" by L. Beytas and G.L. Connors. In *Pulmonary Rehabilitation: Guidelines to Success* (2nd ed.) by J.E. Hodgkin, G.L. Connors, and C.W. Bell (Eds.). Copyright 1992 by J.B. Lippincott.

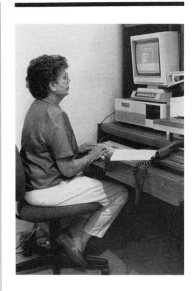

Additionally, a postprogram follow-up questionnaire may be used to gather information relative to compliance with the home program. The information gathered may be tabulated and used for continuous quality improvement. An example of a follow-up questionnaire may be found in Figure 6.1

Essential in the completion of the pulmonary rehabilitation program and subsequent follow-up is the attention paid to providing the primary care physician with information regarding the patient's progress, prescribed home program, and additional information gathered from follow-up activities and questionnaires. Aside from improving patient compliance because of the patient's continued interaction with his or her physician, this insures a continued excellent relationship with the physician and your program.

At the time of program completion, the staff should evaluate whether the patient needs a home health care visit. This visit would include an evaluation of the patient's need for adaptive equipment and other supplies,[14] and an assessment and referral to available community services. A comprehensive pulmonary rehabilitation program needs to have a solid structure. This structure has a foundation that is laid in the initial interview, continues to build during the immediate rehabilitation program, and is finalized with a continued follow-up aftercare program.

The discharge summary documenting the patient's outcomes should be sent to the primary care physician.

Continuous Quality Improvement

A continuous quality improvement (CQI) program, designed to objectively and systematically monitor and evaluate the quality and appropriateness of patient care, is important. It can be used to improve patient care and correct problems identified. The CQI program should conform to current Joint Commission on Accreditation of Healthcare Organizations (JCAHO) requirements as well as the Medicare Conditions of Participation.[15,16]

Figure 6.1
Pulmonary Rehabilitation Program Follow-Up Questionnaire

Name: ______________________________

Evaluation date: ____________________ Response date: ____________________

Your thoughts about your health and quality of life are important to us in helping to determine the effectiveness of the training and exercise components in our pulmonary rehabilitation program. This questionnaire will help us to understand how our program affected you. We appreciate your time and cooperation in answering the questions. Please read each question carefully. Thank you!

Health

1. How would you rate each of the following *now* as compared to *before* you participated in the pulmonary rehabilitation program? (Circle one per line)

A. Shortness of breath	Better	No change	Worse
B. Cough	Less	No change	More
C. Sputum amount	Less	No change	More
D. Sputum consistency	Thinner	No change	Thicker
E. Wheezing	Less	No change	More
F. Swelling of feet/ankles	Less	No change	More
G. Appetite	Better	No change	Worse
H. Sleep	Better	No change	Worse
I. Getting out of the house	More	No change	Less
J. Sexual activity	Better	No change	Worse

2. Have you had any respiratory infections in the past 3 months?

   No Yes If yes, please answer the following:

   a) How many have you had? __________

   b) Did you use an antibiotic for your respiratory infection? __________

   If yes, name the antibiotic used ______________________________

3. Do you smoke? No Yes If yes, how much per day? ____________________

4. Do you drink alcohol? No Yes If yes, how much per day? ____________________

5. How many days have you been hospitalized in the past 3 months? __________

6. List the medications you are currently using:

   ____

   ____

   ____

7. Are you using supplemental oxygen? No Yes If yes, how many hours per day? __________

Work

1. Has there been any change in your work situation since you graduated from the pulmonary rehabilitation program? (Circle one)

   A. No Yes A change in job (explain) ______________________________

B.　No　Yes　Have you quit your job?

C.　No　Yes　Have you reduced the number of hours worked?

D.　No　Yes　Have you increased the number of hours worked?

E.　No　Yes　Have you retired?

2. Has your spouse's working situation changed since you graduated from the pulmonary rehabilitation program?　(Circle one)

A.　No　Yes　Started working?

B.　No　Yes　Stopped working?

Home and family

1. Has there been any change in your living situation since you graduated from the pulmonary rehabilitation program?　(Circle one)

A.　No　Yes　Change in address?　If yes, please write below:

_____

B.　No　Yes　Change in marital status?　If yes, circle one:

　　1) No　Yes　Married

　　2) No　Yes　Divorced

　　3) No　Yes　Death of a spouse

Diet

1. How would you compare your diet (eating habits) *now* as compared to *before* the pulmonary rehabilitation program?　(Circle one)

A.	Food portions	More	No change	Less
B.	Eating whole grains	More	No change	Less
C.	Eating vegetables	More	No change	Less
D.	Eating fruits	More	No change	Less
E.	Eating foods high in fat	More	No change	Less
F.	Drinking fluids	More	No change	Less
G.	Use of salt	More	No change	Less

2. What is your current weight? _____

Exercise

1. How would you rate your exercise (activity) level *now* as compared to *before* the pulmonary rehabilitation program?　(Circle one)

　　　　　　　　More　　　　No change　　　　Less

2. List the type of exercise you do (walk, golf, bicycle, etc.):

_____

3. How many days per week do you exercise? _____

4. How many minutes do you exercise on these days? _____

Note. "Pulmonary Rehabilitation Program Follow-Up Questionnaire" is reprinted courtesy of the Pulmonary Rehabilitation Program at St. Helena Hospital, Napa Valley, CA.

CQI is a process of continuing improvement in all areas of pulmonary rehabilitation. By knowing what the patient community wants, we can focus on optimizing care by preventing problems instead of dealing with errors or complaints when they occur. A patient's evaluation of the total program upon completion is helpful to determine weaknesses and patient perceptions. This information is then used in the CQI program for pulmonary rehabilitation.

The CQI program being implemented by JCAHO looks at assuring quality care.[17] W. Edwards Deming is considered the "guru" of CQI.[18] The major principles of CQI are to further the mission of the organization through the total effort and commitment of every member of the organization. The process must be understood by all; and a search for continuous improvement cannot be based on fear or frustration. The CQI program looks at *outcomes*, assessing the end results of care, the goal being to enhance understanding of the effectiveness of various interventions, to disseminate national standards or practice guidelines to caregivers, and to provide data to the "publics" of health care: the patient, payor, and provider. The outcome movement will reduce variation and by 1993 will be a part of JCAHO. Clinical indicators are the tools from which outcomes are determined.[19-22] It is important for the pulmonary rehabilitation team to be in tune with the focus of CQI, outcomes, and clinical indicators. The movement has already started in the health care arena, and pulmonary rehabilitation can reap the benefits of that work.

A CQI program looks at *outcomes*, assessing the end results of care.

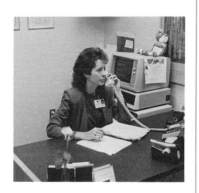

Conclusion

An important aspect of follow-up is the long-term team support of the patient's "new" lifestyle. This is important to the long-term success and outcomes of the pulmonary rehabilitation patient. A CQI program is important for monitoring the pulmonary rehabilitation program and may be used for increasing the public's knowledge of pulmonary disease and rehabilitation. For comprehensive pulmonary rehabilitation to occur, thorough follow-up is necessary. It is one of the essential components of pulmonary rehabilitation.

References

1. Sneider R, O'Malley JA, Kahn M. Trends in pulmonary rehabilitation at Eisenhower Medical Center: our 11 years experience (1976-1987). *J Cardiop Rehab.* 1988;11:453-461.
2. Hodgkin JE. Prognosis in chronic obstructive pulmonary disease. *Clin Chest Med.* 1990;11(3):555-569.
3. Burns MR, Sherman B, Madison R, Kao D, Petty TL. Pulmonary rehabilitation outcome. *The Jr for Resp Care Practitioners.* Iowa City, Iowa: 1989;2(1):25-30.
4. Anthonisen NR, Wright EC, Hodgkin JE. Prognosis in chronic obstructive pulmonary disease. *Am Rev Respir Dis.* 1986;133:14-20.
5. Moser KM, Bokinsky GE, Savage RT, Archibald CJ, Hansen PR. Results of a comprehensive rehabilitation program: physiologic and

functional effects on patients with chronic obstructive pulmonary disease. *Arch Intern Med.* 1980;140:1596-1601.

6. Ries AL. Pulmonary rehabilitation. In: Fishman AP, ed. *Pulmonary Diseases and Disorders.* 2nd ed. New York, NY: McGraw-Hill Book Co; 1988:1325-1331.

7. Petty TL, Nett LM, Finigan MM, Brink GA, Corsello PR. A comprehensive care program for chronic airway obstruction: methods and preliminary evaluation of symptomatic and functional improvement. *Ann Intern Med.* 1969;70:1109-1120.

8. Lertzman MM, Cherniack RM. Rehabilitation of patients with chronic obstructive pulmonary disease. *Am Rev Respir Dis.* 1976;114:1145-1165.

9. Bebout DE, Hodgkin JE, Zorn EG, Yee AR, Sammer EA. Clinical and physiological outcomes of a university-hospital pulmonary rehabilitation program. *Respir Care.* 1983;28:1468-1473.

10. Mall RW, Medeiros M. Objective evaluation of results of a pulmonary rehabilitation program in a community hospital. *Chest.* 1988;94:1156-1160.

11. Holden DA, Stelmach KD, Curtis PS, Beck GJ, Stoller JK. The impact of a rehabilitation program on functional status of patients with chronic lung disease. *Respir Care.* 1990;35(4):332-341.

12. Make BJ. Pulmonary rehabilitation: what are the outcomes. *Respir Care.* 1990;35(4):329-331. Editorial.

13. Fishman DB, Petty TL. Physical, symptomatic, and psychological improvement in patients receiving comprehensive care for chronic airway obstruction. *J Chronic Dis.* 1971;24:775-785.

14. McPherson SP. *Respiratory Home Care Equipment.* Iowa City, Iowa: Kendall/Hunt Publishing Co;1988:1-120.

15. *Accreditation Manual for Hospitals.* Chicago, Ill: Joint Commission for Accreditation of Hospital Organizations; 1991.

16. Hall LK. Quality assurance in cardiac and pulmonary rehabilitation. *J Cardiop Rehab.* 1990;10:117-119. Editorial.

17. Roberts JS, Schyue PM. From QA to QI: the views and role of the joint commission. *The Quality Letter.* May 1990:9-12.

18. Lynn ML, Osborn DP. Deming's quality principles: a health care application. *Hospitals and Health Services Administration.* 1991;36(1):7-16.

19. Agency for Health Care Policy and Research. US Dept of Health and Human Services. *Allied Health Perspectives on Guideline Development.* Washington, DC: November 1990;OM91-0507.

20. Fletcher RH, Fletcher SW. Clinical practice guidelines. *Ann Intern Med.* 1990;113(9):645-646. Editorial.

21. Joint Commissions Agenda for Change. Characteristics of clinical indicators. *QRB.* November 1989:330-339.

22. McGuire LB. A long run for a short jump: understanding clinical guidelines. *Ann Intern Med.* 1989;113:705-708.

Chapter 7

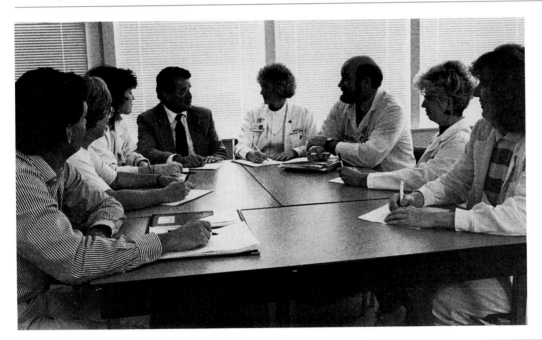

Program Management

Qualified health care personnel, working in conjunction with the patient's primary care physician and program medical director, provide the services and strategies for successful rehabilitation of the pulmonary patient.[1] The number of team members and their professional backgrounds will vary considerably from one facility to another. It is not necessary for every member of a multidisciplinary team to assess each patient; however, the collective knowledge, skills, and clinical experiences of the professional staff should reflect the multidisciplinary expertise necessary to achieve the desired program and patient goals.[2,3] Team communication and interaction are vital to successful rehabilitation of the pulmonary patient.

Team communication and interaction are vital to successful rehabilitation of the pulmonary patient.

Team Responsibilities

To achieve patient and program goals, the rehabilitation team should have the knowledge and technical skills necessary to carry out the following responsibilities:

1. Assess patients
2. Determine realistic patient goals
3. Coordinate and provide treatment programs

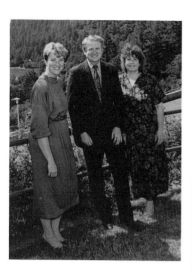

4. Evaluate patient progress
5. Document services provided
6. Plan and recommend continued self-care program for the patient and her or his primary care physician

Team Structure

A pulmonary rehabilitation team at the very least should include a medical director and a designated coordinator. Team members may be full- or part-time and may include both licensed and nonlicensed health care professionals. It is very helpful to have at least one full-time team member (usually the coordinator).

The pulmonary rehabilitation team may include any or all of the following[4]:

- Medical director
- Respiratory therapist or technician
- Registered or licensed vocational nurse
- Physical therapist
- Exercise physiologist
- Occupational therapist
- Pulmonary laboratory technologist
- Dietitian
- Pharmacist
- Social worker
- Chaplain or pastoral care associate
- Recreational therapist
- Clinical psychologist
- Psychiatrist
- Vocational rehabilitation counselor
- Speech therapist
- Biofeedback technician
- Home care personnel
- Business office representative

The American Thoracic Society (ATS) official position statement on pulmonary rehabilitation states, "Pulmonary rehabilitation programs may be of different sizes and configurations. All allied health professionals may not be represented on every team in every hospital; however, all services listed in the ATS statement must be available and provided by someone. Although every patient with COPD may not require all these services, selected patients may need them all"[2] (see Appendix B).

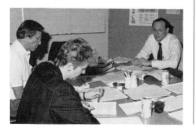

Team Conference

Regular team conferences enhance team communication and necessary follow-up of patient goals. The components of a team conference include a short description of the patient's history and physical exam, each team member's patient assessment and target/problem areas evaluated, and a determination of treatment modalities and necessary discharge plans. Documentation of the conference, and its placement in the patient's medical chart, are important to show team progress toward the determined patient goals. Each program's policies should determine the inclusion of the program director's and medical director's signatures on the document.

Personnel Qualifications

All personnel should be trained in basic life-support techniques. The following are the minimum guidelines for ''core'' personnel.

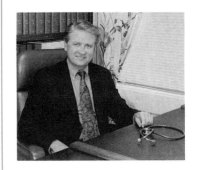

Medical Directors

The medical director should be a licensed physician with an interest in pulmonary rehabilitation and knowledge of pulmonary function and exercise testing. The role of the medical director varies in different programs. He or she often functions as an administrator, diagnostician, clinician, educator, and research coordinator.

Program Director/Coordinator

The program director or coordinator should be trained in a health-related profession and have clinical experience and expertise in the care of pulmonary patients.[6] She or he should understand the philosophy and goals of pulmonary rehabilitation and be knowledgeable in administration, marketing, and education.

Other Team Members

At least one team member should have national certification or state licensure in a health-related specialty (e.g., respiratory care, nursing, or physical therapy). This person may or may not be the program coordinator. All team members should have training or experience in working with the pulmonary patient. Each team member is responsible for his or her specific specialty but should also be able to work as part of a multidisciplinary team. All individuals should contribute to developing and implementing program goals and strategies. The ability to communicate effectively with patients, colleagues, and the general public is an important attribute.

Facilities

The facilities and equipment used for pulmonary rehabilitation should meet state and federal safety code standards. Sufficient space should be available for the multiple services provided. The physical area can vary greatly depending upon program structure, needs, and resources. A positive environment is important in attaining program and patient goals. In addition, pulmonary rehabilitation programs often serve as the first contact for patients and the general public with the health care facility. Therefore, such programs can play an important role in the public relations and marketing plans of the parent organization.

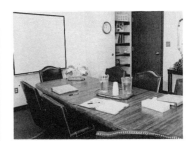

Some specific considerations for a pulmonary rehabilitation environment are these:

- Adequate and convenient parking
- Access for individuals with disabilities
- Sufficient space for classroom, exercise, clinical, and administrative activities
- Storage space for pulmonary equipment (e.g., oxygen, wheelchairs, walkers, respiratory therapy equipment)
- Bathrooms
- Optimal light, temperature, and ventilation (these are particularly important for pulmonary patients)

Location

As Table 7.1 indicates, pulmonary rehabilitation programs may be conducted in a variety of locations. Typically, programs are located in the inpatient or outpatient areas of hospitals. Clinics, comprehensive outpatient rehabilitation facilities (CORFs), YMCAs and YWCAs, Jewish Community Centers, and a myriad of other settings provide potential sites for rehabilitation programs. The essential requirements in selecting a site are accessibility for the patient, an environment conducive

Pulmonary rehabilitation programs may be conducted in a variety of locations.

Table 7.1   Location Options for Pulmonary Rehabilitation Programs

Inpatient care
   Acute care during hospitalization
   Transitional care unit
   Rehabilitation hospital

Outpatient care
   Outpatient hospital setting
   Physician office
   Clinic setting
   Residential outpatient facility
   Comprehensive Outpatient Rehabilitation
   Facility (CORF)
   Shared facility with other rehabilitation programs

Alternate sites
   Storefront
   Home residence
   Fitness center or spa
   Wellness center
   Senior citizen center
   Local high school or community college
   Adult education center
   Places of worship
   Club meeting halls

Note. Reprinted with permission from "Organization and Management of a Pulmonary Rehabilitation Program" by L. Beytas and G.L. Connors. In *Pulmonary Rehabilitation: Guidelines to Success* (2nd ed.) by J.E. Hodgkin, G.L. Connors, and C.W. Bell (Eds.). Copyright 1992 by J.B. Lippincott.

to good health, and appropriate medical and emergency supervision. Additionally, the site must be able to provide all of the components of a comprehensive rehabilitation program from assessment, patient training, exercise, and psychosocial intervention to follow-up care.

Group Size and Schedule

Pulmonary rehabilitation programs are most commonly conducted in small groups of approximately four to six patients or one on one. Programs may also be arranged for individual patients. Regardless of program size or design, it should be individualized to meet each patient's goals and needs. Program schedules will vary according to staff, facilities, resources, and patient needs. It is difficult to set specific guidelines; however, a typical program may include 30 to 40 hours over a 4- to 8-week period. Program schedules vary among facilities due to patients' degrees of impairment, limitations, ages, and (possibly) job schedules. A typical pulmonary rehabilitation program includes patient training and exercise sessions each time the program meets after the initial evaluations are completed. See Table 7.2 for a sample outpatient program schedule. Patients' specific needs should be reflected in the patients' schedules.

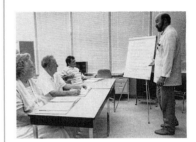

Table 7.2 Sample of a 5-Week Outpatient Pulmonary Rehabilitation Program Schedule

Week	Tuesday	Thursday	Friday
1	1:00-2:00 Orientation to PR 2:00-3:00 Breathing retraining 3:00-4:30 Introduction to exercise training	1:00-2:00 Inhaler instruction 2:00-3:00 Support group 3:00-4:30 Supervised exercise training	1:00-2:30 Supervised exercise training
2	1:00-2:00 The respiratory system: structure and function 2:00-3:00 Coping with chronic disease 3:00-4:30 Supervised exercise training	1:00-2:00 Medications 2:00-3:00 Respiratory muscle training 3:00-4:30 Supervised exercise training	1:00-2:30 Supervised exercise training
3	1:00-2:00 Medical testing and evaluation review 2:00-3:00 Respiratory equipment 3:00-4:30 Supervised exercise training	1:00-2:00 Panic control/relaxation techniques 2:00-3:00 Time and energy conservation 3:00-4:30 Supervised exercise training	1:00-2:30 Supervised exercise training
4	1:00-2:00 Self-assessment techniques 2:00-3:00 Nutrition and the lungs 3:00-4:30 Supervised exercise training	1:00-2:00 Importance of exercise 2:00-3:00 Community resources 3:00-4:30 Supervised exercise training	1:00-2:30 Supervised exercise training
5	1:00-2:00 Preventing infection 2:00-3:00 Traveling with lung disease 3:00-4:30 Supervised exercise training	1:00-2:00 Environmental lung factors 2:00-3:00 Intimate relations 3:00-4:30 Supervised exercise training	1:00-2:30 Supervised exercise training 2:30-3:30 Home recommendation 3:30-4:30 Graduation

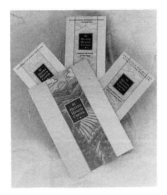

Marketing Pulmonary Rehabilitation

Program success depends upon consumer awareness, which is accomplished through developing a marketing strategy and program. Marketing is not just advertising; it is an organized and structured process that determines (1) who the customer is—patients, patients' families, and physicians, and (2) what the customer needs—programs consisting of assessment, training, exercise, psychosocial intervention, and follow-up. From this information a marketing plan is created and put into action to ensure program success. Numerous texts include entire chapters devoted to marketing strategies and plans.[7-9] The most successful marketing team in all programs is the frontline team that interfaces with the patient. Also contributing to their success are the activities that the rehabilitation team does with the community (e.g., newspaper, TV, and radio interviews; wellness fairs; and speeches to nonprofit groups such as the Elks, Kiwanis, and chamber of commerce meetings).

Customers, physicians, patients, family members, providers of goods and services, buyers, payors, and technical-assist people become target markets and potential publics. Each plan involves assessing and auditing the external environment, looking at the internal system for providing the product, defining the product, pricing the product, and finally, planning for promotion of the product. Implementation is the final phase of a marketing plan. Marketing plans often fail because homework is not done relative to the following:

1. Is there a need for the program in this market area?
2. What are the consumer needs relative to this program?
3. Will the physicians support the program with referrals?
4. Can we provide what is needed?

An example of a national marketing idea that may then spin off to local programs is the utilization of National Pulmonary Rehabilitation Week. This occurs every year in the first week of spring and is promoted by the American Association of Cardiovascular and Pulmonary Rehabilitation (AACVPR). Figure 7.1 is an example of a proclamation

Figure 7.1
Proclamation for National Rehabilitation Week

Whereas, lung disease constitutes a critical, social, and economic health problem in the United States; and

Whereas, pulmonary rehabilitation is a vital component of comprehensive quality care of the lung patient, but both the public and medical communities are generally unaware of its physical, emotional, and economic benefits; and

Whereas, the incidence of lung disease can be reduced through earlier detection, treatment, prevention, and rehabilitation; and

Whereas, the establishment of a special week each year to promote lung disease awareness, prevention, and rehabilitation will greatly assist in decreasing its incidence;

Now, therefore, I, _____, do hereby proclaim the first week of spring as Pulmonary Rehabilitation Week in our community, and urge all citizens to generously support this most worthy effort.

Note. Reprinted with permission from "Marketing the Pulmonary Rehabilitation Program" by G.L. Connors, S. Schnell-Hobbs, and W. Syvertsen. In *Pulmonary Rehabilitation: Guidelines to Success* (2nd ed.) by J.E. Hodgkin, G.L. Connors, and C.W. Bell (Eds.). Copyright 1992 by J.B. Lippincott.

used to promote community awareness of lung disease and rehabilitation. The AACVPR can help individual programs promote this day by providing individual marketing kits. It is essential to view and market the pulmonary rehabilitation program from a global perspective, remembering that it is preventive as well as therapeutic.

Documentation and Reimbursement

Documentation is important for successful rehabilitation of the pulmonary patient and for reimbursement.[10] Accurate and thorough charting facilitates effective communication among various team members and helps staff monitor each patient's progress toward her or his goals. It is also useful for continued quality improvement (CQI) and for communicating with third-party payors.

Basic requirements for documentation for pulmonary rehabilitation include these:

- Physician orders for the program treatment modalities
- Patient assessment and delineation of patient goals and target areas for treatment
- Daily treatment record
- Team conferences after the initial assessment and at regular intervals during the program
- Recommendations for a home self-care program

An individual patient chart is a convenient way to organize documentation. Specific forms should adhere to requirements of the medical records department of the institution. Charting relates the patient response to the treatment given. The format for charting may vary, but it should always refer to the specific problem or target area being treated.

Charting forms may include but are not limited to the following:

- Flow sheets—for supervised exercise, symptom management instruction, medications, dyspnea response to ADLs
- Individualized progress notes

Content
Charts should include individual patient response to program interventions and changes noted in patient function observed by pulmonary rehabilitation team members. Progress toward the patient's rehabilitation goals and outcomes must be documented.

Format
Charts should include narrative commentary or four types of data: subjective, objective, assessment, and plan (SOAP).

(S) *Subjective* data documents the patient's verbalized feelings or complaints.

(O) *Objective* data documents measurable responses and observations of the rehabilitation staff.

(A) *Assessment* data documents results of the intervention as determined by the provider.

(P) *Plan* data documents the next steps in the rehabilitation intervention based on patient performance as documented in the assessment data.[11]

Documentation is important for successful rehabilitation and for reimbursement.

Charting forms may include flow sheets, individualized progress notes, periodic progress updates, and discharge records.

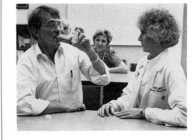

Discharge records should include a medication record, home exercise recommendations, pulmonary rehabilitation recommendations, and a discharge summary.

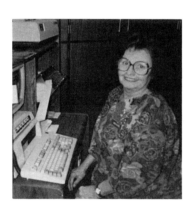

Frequency

Documentation is needed for each intervention/treatment/training of the rehabilitation patient.

- Periodic progress notations—documents achievement toward meeting the patient's individualized program goals
- Discharge records
    a. Medication record—instructs patient on physician's medication orders.
    b. Home exercise recommendations—instructs patient in progressive home exercise program and guidelines for change.
    c. Pulmonary rehabilitation recommendations—instructs patient in self-care maintenance and symptom management techniques.
    d. Discharge summary—documents interventions and patient progress in the rehabilitation program. Copies of diagnostic studies performed are commonly included in this report.

It is important to carefully follow billing and charting requirements of third-party payors to insure appropriate reimbursement for services rendered. Program directors and staff should be familiar with current Health Care Financing Administration (HCFA) guidelines and policies pertaining to pulmonary rehabilitation. These are frequently followed by other third-party payors. There are differences in how reimbursement guidelines are applied in different regions by various intermediaries and third-party payors.[12,13]

It is also recommended that the program have a close liaison with the business office to insure that billing information is complete and accurate and that problems with reimbursement are addressed promptly and effectively.

A close working relationship with the medical records department is also helpful to insure that complete records are kept and made available for third-party payor audit or other review.

Conclusion

A successful pulmonary rehabilitation program combines effective management techniques and structure; a supportive and actively participating medical director; and a dedicated, knowledgeable, and enthusiastic program director. Motivation and inspiration from the director along with good leadership and team-building techniques affect the success of the entire pulmonary rehabilitation staff.

Location, program schedules, and equipment may vary as the needs of the patients, families, and community dictate. Several regulatory agencies such as the Joint Commission on Accreditation of Healthcare Organizations (JCAHO) require current documentation for each patient with regard to program goals, progress, expected outcomes, and final outcomes. This documentation facilitates effective communication among team members as the patient proceeds through the rehabilitation program, and it is also necessary for reimbursement.

Marketing the program is essential from the beginning. Market planning assists in designing the program by providing analysis of the customers and their needs and the community within which the program will exist. A strategic marketing plan will also enhance operations and assist in making plans for future expansions.

Finally, location, structure, marketing, record keeping, and all of the other program components are only as successful as the people who put them into operation. Successful pulmonary rehabilitation programs develop a team of specialized individuals who come together with common goals of enhancing the lives of the unique and challenging group of people with lung disease.

Successful programs develop a team of specialized individuals who come together with common goals of enhancing the lives of people with lung disease.

References

1. Maddox SE, Selecky PA, Barry MS, McLean DL. Organization and structure of a pulmonary rehabilitation program. In: Hodgkin JE, Zorn EG, Connors GL, eds. *Pulmonary Rehabilitation: Guidelines to Success.* Boston, Mass: Butterworth; 1984:9-25.
2. Hodgkin JE, Farrell MJ, Gibson SR, et al. Pulmonary rehabilitation: official American Thoracic Society statement. *Amer Rev Respir Dis.* 1981;124:663-666.
3. Hodgkin JE, Gray LS, Connors GL, eds. *Pulmonary Rehabilitation and Continuing Care.* Special issue. *Resp Care.* 1983;28:1419-1528.
4. Hodgkin JE, Asmus RM, Connors GA. Pulmonary rehabilitation: designing a program that works. *J Respir Dis.* 1987;8(12):55-68.
5. Yee AR, Hodgkin JE. The role of the medical director. In: Hodgkin JE, Zorn EG, Connors GL, eds. *Pulmonary Rehabilitation: Guidelines to Success.* Boston, Mass: Butterworth; 1984:23-25.
6. Mall RW, Medeiros M. Objective evaluation of results of a pulmonary rehabilitation program in a community hospital. *Chest.* 1988;94:1156-1160.
7. Kotler P, Clark RN. *Marketing for Health Care Organizations.* Englewood Cliffs, NJ: Prentice Hall; 1987.
8. Cottle DW. *Client-Centered Service: How to Keep Them Coming Back for More.* New York, NY: Wiley & Sons; 1990.
9. Kotler P, Andreasen AR. *Strategic Marketing for Non-Profit Organizations.* 3rd ed. Englewood Cliffs, NJ: Prentice Hall; 1987.
10. Bunch D. Pulmonary rehabilitation directors struggle with reimbursement. *AARC Times.* 1991;15(7):48-49.
11. Fink JB, Fink AK. *The Respiratory Therapist as Manager.* Chicago, Ill: Year Book Medical Publishing Inc; 1986:372-373.
12. Elkousy NM, Komorowski D, Foto M, et al. Outpatient pulmonary rehabilitation: a Medicare fiscal intermediary's viewpoint. *J Cardiop Rehab.* 1988;8(11):492-497.
13. Task Force on Financing Quality Health Care for Persons with Diabetes. *Third-party Reimbursement for Diabetes Outpatient Education. A Manual for Health Care Professions.* Developed by the American Diabetes Assoc Inc; 1986.

Position Paper of the American Association of Cardiovascular and Pulmonary Rehabilitation: Scientific Basis of Pulmonary Rehabilitation

Andrew L. Ries, MD

Scientific Basis of Pulmonary Rehabilitation

I. Epidemiology of COPD

II. Definition and Overview of Pulmonary Rehabilitation
  A. Patient Selection
  B. Patient Evaluation
    1. Medical Evaluation
    2. Psychosocial Assessment

III. Benefits
  A. General Benefits
    1. Hospitalizations/Medical Resources
    2. Quality of Life/Symptoms
    3. Pulmonary Function Tests
    4. Survival
    5. Occupational Changes
    6. Long-Term Follow-Up
  B. Specific Components
    1. Education

2. Respiratory and Chest Physiotherapy
  a. Bronchial Hygiene
  b. Breathing Training Techniques
    (1) Diaphragmatic Breathing
    (2) Pursed-Lips Breathing
  c. Oxygen

3. Psychosocial Support
  a. Relaxation Training

4. Exercise
  a. Benefits—Controlled Studies
  b. Benefits—Uncontrolled Studies
  c. Prescription
  d. Exercise-Induced Hypoxemia
  e. Other Types of Exercise
    (1) Upper Extremity
    (2) Ventilatory Muscle

The AACVPR thanks the following individuals for their contributions in reviewing this position paper: Michael J. Belman, MD, Eileen Hanafin Breslin, RN, DNSc, Neil F. Gordon, MD, PhD, MPH, John E. Hodgkin, MD, Donald A. Mahler, MD, and William P. Marley, PhD.

Epidemiology of COPD

In the latter part of the 20th century, with the declining importance of acute infectious diseases and the progressively aging population, the greatest challenges to Western medicine are increasingly focused on chronic conditions and their associated disabilities.[188]

The chronic obstructive pulmonary diseases (COPD), including emphysema and chronic bronchitis, are characterized by chronic airway obstruction and reduction in expiratory airflow. These diseases, major causes of death and disability, have increased in prevalence dramatically in the 20th century. In the United States in the 1980s, these diseases ranked as the fifth leading cause of death and accounted for approximately 4% of all deaths.[76,77,104] In addition, they are cited as contributory causes about one and one half times as frequently (e.g., in 1983, COPD was the primary cause of 62,000 deaths and contributed to an additional 90,000+ deaths).[76] Among causes of death for individuals 55 to 74 years of age, COPD ranks third among men and fourth among women.

In contrast to other major diseases, death rates from COPD in the United States have increased rapidly in recent years. For instance, from 1970 to 1980, death rates from coronary heart disease, the number one cause of death, decreased nearly 30% while deaths from COPD increased more than 60%.[172,173] Since 1980, these trends have continued, particularly among men older than 75 years and in women older than 45 years of age (i.e., rates have stabilized in men younger than 75 years).[77,39] In Great Britain, four fifths of all deaths attributable to COPD occur in individuals age 65 or older.[188] In addition, there has been an increasing proportion of disease and deaths among women with the male:female ratio decreasing from 4.30 in 1970 to 2.36 in 1980.[172] In other countries, death rates from COPD are more variable; in general, they are increasing in women in developed countries.[125] However, it is unclear whether these international differences are real or represent various methods of data collection.

The true prevalence of these diseases is unknown but has been reported from 10% to up to more than 30% of the adult population depending on the population studied and definition of disease.[62,76,116,188,190] The natural history of COPD spans several decades and has been associated primarily with cigarette smoking as the major risk factor.[51,62] Additional risk factors include air pollution (atmospheric, domestic, and occupational), childhood respiratory infections, and, possibly, passive smoking.[30,42,51,190] Asthma is also an obstructive disease of the airways that overlaps considerably with COPD in its chronic forms; therefore, asthma may also be an important risk factor contributing to the development of COPD.[31,190]

Although smoking is the major risk factor for development of COPD, the majority of cigarette smokers do not develop clinical manifestations of obstructive lung disease. Typically, these diseases develop insidiously and, because of the large reserve in lung function, do not produce significant symptoms or come to medical attention until at an advanced stage.[62] Many patients with mild to moderate disease have few symptoms and are undiagnosed. Therefore, official health statistics significantly underreport the number of cases. On the other hand, when the disease is recognized later in life, lung function is often severely compromised and the disease process may be largely irreversible. Survival rates for patients with diagnosed COPD are severely reduced with approximate survivals of 50% at 5 years and 25% at 10 years.[180]

Problems of morbidity and the resultant disability from these diseases are also significant. In the United States, COPD is second only to coronary heart disease in the number of patients receiving Social Security disability payments for severe disease (estimated at more than 500,000 patients). Respiratory illnesses, often from acute respiratory infections, are the most common cause of loss time from work. In addition, the effects of respiratory infections are much more serious among patients with underlying chronic lung disease, many of whom are undiagnosed, unrecognized, and in older age groups. Data from the National Ambulatory Medical Care Survey in 1985 indicate that for the age group from 55 to 84 years, COPD and allied conditions were responsible for 16.4% of physician office visits for men and 12.5% for women.[77] Data from the National Hospital Discharge Survey in 1986 indicate that COPD and allied conditions were the first listed condition in the discharge summary in 923,000 hospitalizations; this represents 1.3% of hospital discharges for men and 0.9% for women in patients aged 55 to 84 years.[77] Approximately half of these discharges were for asthma and the other half for the various categories of

"COPD." The estimated costs for these illnesses are enormous, estimated at more than $26 billion in 1982.[104]

In Great Britain, it has been estimated that chronic lung diseases are responsible for more than half a million periods of sickness absence from work per year (10% of recorded working days lost due to sickness) and for 10% of hospital bed occupancy.[49,188] Also, estimates indicate that respiratory diseases account for 25% of general practitioner consultations.[85]

Definition and Overview of Pulmonary Rehabilitation

In general, the goals of medical therapy are to relieve symptoms, improve functional status, and enhance quality of life. Standard medical treatment is important in alleviating symptoms of COPD, particularly the distressing symptom of breathlessness (dyspnea).[6] However, many patients, families, and physicians are left to cope with the problems of a chronic, largely irreversible disease process associated with disabling symptoms that limit functional capacity and impair quality of life. The medical attitude for symptomatic treatment is often nihilistic, directed toward writing prescriptions, and conditioned by the attitude that "nothing more can be done." Survival in patients with COPD is related to age and degree of pulmonary impairment (i.e., FEV_1); however, when adjusted for these variables, the patient's exercise tolerance and perceived physical disability may also be important predictors of mortality.[8]

Pulmonary rehabilitation programs for patients with chronic lung diseases are well established as a means of providing a comprehensive approach to enhance standard medical therapy to control and alleviate symptoms and optimize functional capacity.[5,6,49,80,82,84,98,105,110,121,138,146] The primary goal of these programs is to restore the patient to the highest possible level of independent function. This goal may be accomplished by helping patients to become more knowledgeable about their disease, more actively involved in their own health care, more independent in performing daily care activities, and therefore, less dependent on family, friends, health professionals, and expensive medical resources. Rather than focusing solely on reversing a chronic, progressive disease process,

rehabilitation programs attempt to reverse the patient's disability from disease.

In 1974, the American College of Chest Physicians' Committee on Pulmonary Rehabilitation adopted the following definition:

> Pulmonary rehabilitation may be defined as an art of medical practice wherein an individually tailored, multidisciplinary program is formulated which through accurate diagnosis, therapy, emotional support, and education, stabilizes or reverses both the physio- and psychopathology of pulmonary diseases and attempts to return the patient to the highest possible functional capacity allowed by his pulmonary handicap and overall life situation.[5]

This definition focuses on three important features of successful rehabilitation programs:

- *Individual:* Patients with disabling COPD require individual assessment of their needs, individual attention, and a program designed to meet realistic individual goals.
- *Multidisciplinary:* Pulmonary rehabilitation programs provide access to information from a variety of health care disciplines, which is integrated by experienced staff into a comprehensive, cohesive program tailored to the needs of each patient.
- *Attention to Physio- and Psychopathology:* To be successful, pulmonary rehabilitation programs must pay attention to psychological and social problems as well as helping to optimize medical therapy to improve lung function.

Successful pulmonary rehabilitation programs are typically provided by a multidisciplinary team of health care professionals. The responsibilities of team members generally cross disciplines; team makeup may vary depending on the resources and availability of expertise in the specific health care setting. The skills and abilities required of team members have been delineated.[99]

Within this general framework, successful pulmonary rehabilitation programs have been established in various settings (e.g., inpatient or outpatient, hospital- or practice-based and with different formats).[17,70,74,84,98,111,121,138,186] There are distinct advantages and disadvantages of both inpatient and outpatient programs that have been elucidated.[70,98] For instance, inpatient management, particularly in the early phases of rehabilitation, offers distinct advantages for patients with more severe disease.[93,98,121] On the other hand, outpatient programs may be more appropriate for other patients. The particular structure of a given program depends on a number of factors including patient characteristics, costs, available staff and resources, and social considerations. The key to success in any program is often a dedicated and enthusiastic staff who are familiar with the problems of pulmonary patients and who can relate well to and motivate them. Since many of the patients are elderly, program staff should be particularly sensitive to the needs and problems of older individuals.[131]

Although pulmonary rehabilitation programs have been developed primarily for patients with COPD, these programs may also be useful for patients with other pulmonary diseases.[65,70]

Patient Selection

An important factor in the success of pulmonary rehabilitation is the appropriate selection of patients. Any patient with symptomatic chronic lung disease is a candidate for a pulmonary rehabilitation program.[5,48] Appropriate patients are those who recognize that they have symptoms due to lung disease, perceive some impairment or disability related to that disease, and are motivated to be active participants in their own care to improve their health status. Patients with mild disease may not recognize their disease or may not perceive their problem as severe enough to warrant a comprehensive care program. On the other hand, patients with severe disease without reserve in lung function may be too limited to benefit significantly. Resting hypercapnia alone should not be considered an indication of too severe lung disease. Foster and coworkers reported that hypercapnic patients improved exercise tolerance and achieved benefits from pulmonary rehabilitation similar to the eucapnic patients.[64]

Other factors are also important in evaluating patients as candidates for pulmonary rehabilitation. The role of the rehabilitation program is typically to act in support of the patient, family, and primary care physician and not to provide direct medical care. Pulmonary rehabilitation is not a first-line mode of therapy for COPD. Therefore, patients should generally be stabilized on standard medical therapy before beginning a program. The assessment and treatment plan then can be based on the patient's optimal baseline level of function.

Patients should not have other disabling or unstable conditions that would limit their ability to participate fully in rehabilitation activities. These include, but are not limited to, unstable heart disease, psychiatric illness, or concurrent evaluation for a potentially serious health problem.

The ideal patient for pulmonary rehabilitation, then, is one with moderate to moderately severe lung disease who is stable on standard medical therapy, not distracted or limited by other serious or unstable medical conditions, willing and able to learn about his/her disease, and motivated to devote the time and effort necessary to benefit from a comprehensive care program.

Patient Evaluation

The initial step in evaluating patients for pulmonary rehabilitation programs is a patient interview that thoroughly reviews the patient's medical history and also evaluates psychosocial problems and needs.[5,48] Communication and cooperation with the primary care physician is important in this effort. Care and attention in this initial evaluation provides the foundation to help the patient select appropriate individual goals compatible with patient, family, and physician expectations and the program's objectives.

Medical Evaluation

The patient's medical history should be reviewed thoroughly to characterize and stage severity of the patient's lung disease and to identify other medical problems that might preclude or delay participation in the program. Pertinent laboratory data may include available pulmonary function and exercise tests, arterial blood gases, chest radiographs, electrocardiogram, and blood counts, chemistries, and theophylline level. Additional diagnostic testing then can be planned as needed.

To plan an appropriate program for each patient, it is important to have accurate, current information. The complexity of diagnostic testing performed depends on the individual patient and the facilities available.

Pulmonary function testing helps to characterize and quantify impairment resulting from the patient's lung disease. Spirometry and lung volume measurements are most useful and can be supplemented with other tests such as diffusing capacity, airway resistance, respiratory muscle strength and endurance, or other parameters as needed.[45,189]

Exercise testing is generally necessary to assess the patient's exercise tolerance and to evaluate possible blood gas changes (hypoxemia or hypercapnia) with exercise. This may also help to uncover other coexisting diseases that are common in elderly patients (e.g., heart disease). Other unstable or untreated diseases may contribute to the patient's symptoms or potentially interfere with the rehabilitation effort.[48] The exercise test can also be used to establish a safe and appropriate prescription for subsequent training.[22,78,147]

Maximal exercise tolerance of patients with moderate to severe COPD may be limited by their breathing capacity and/or fatigue of deconditioned muscles. Simple pulmonary function tests such as spirometry can be used to estimate a patient's capacity for sustained breathing (maximum ventilation) during physical activity or exercise. The forced expiratory volume in one second (FEV_1) is the most useful parameter in this regard. However, although the pulmonary function test measurements can be used to provide a rough estimate of a patient's maximum work capacity, the exercise tolerance of many COPD patients will depend considerably on an individual's perception and tolerance of the subjective symptom of breathlessness (dyspnea).[147] In one study of 160 patients with COPD, Jones and coworkers found that the measurement of general health status using the Sickness Impact Profile correlated better with the 6-minute walking distance than any of the spirometric measurements.[94]

Many patients with COPD are physically inactive and deconditioned due to their limited lung function and fear of dyspnea. Therefore, it is important to exercise patients to assess each patient's current level of function and tolerance for limiting symptoms (i.e., dyspnea and muscle fatigue). This assessment is best made using the type of exercise that will be employed in training (e.g., treadmill testing for a walking exercise training program); however, test results from one type of exercise (e.g., cycle ergometer) can be translated to similar forms of exercise (e.g., walking).[152] Variables measured and/or monitored during testing should include workload, heart rate, electrocardiogram, arterial oxygenation, and symptoms. Other measurements such as minute ventilation or expired gas analysis to calculate variables such as oxygen consumption (VO_2) may be performed, depending on the interest and expertise of referring physicians, program staff, and laboratory personnel. Exercise testing protocols also should take into account the considerable variations in test results in stable patients with COPD and the normal improvement that may be seen with repeat testing, particularly in patients who are unused to physical activity.[124]

Measurement of arterial blood gases at rest and during exercise is important because of the frequently unexpected and unpredictable occurrence of exercise-induced hypoxemia.[151] Blood gas sampling during exercise adds a significant degree of complexity to testing. Noninvasive techniques, such as cutaneous oximetry measurements of arterial oxygen saturation, are useful for continuous monitoring but should not be relied on for precise assessment of arterial oxygenation because of their limited accuracy (e.g., confidence limits for measurement of arterial oxygen saturation by cutaneous oximetry = ± 4 to 5% saturation).[150]

Psychosocial Assessment

Successful rehabilitation requires attention not only to physical problems but also to psychological and social problems. Since COPD is typically a silent disease in the early stages, patients and families are generally unaware of the chronic, progressive nature of the disease and unfamiliar with appropriate coping strategies. Patients with COPD develop a number of psychosocial problems as they struggle to deal with symptoms they do not understand.[1,57,58,69,113,140,157] These problems are particularly difficult for older individuals, who must often cope with loss of loved ones, friends, self-esteem, and self-worth as well as the physical and physiological changes of aging and disease. Commonly, such patients become depressed, frightened, anxious, and more dependent on others to care for their needs. Psychological status is an important determinant of pulmonary symptoms reported by patients.[53]

Progressive dyspnea is a frightening symptom and may lead to a vicious "fear-dyspnea" cycle: with progressive disease, less exertion results in more dyspnea, which produces more fear and anxiety which, in turn, leads to more dyspnea. Ultimately, the patient avoids any physical activity associated with these unpleasant symptoms of both fear and dyspnea. In the extreme, patients may set up a stationary "command post" from which they rarely venture forth except to seek relief in physicians' offices and hospitals.

To cope with these problems, the initial evaluation should include an assessment of the patient's psychological state (e.g., depression or other psychological tests) and close attention to psychosocial clues during screening interviews (e.g., family and social support, living arrangement, activities of daily living, hobbies, employment potential).[58] Cognitive impairment, which may limit the patient's ability to participate, must be recognized. Spouses, family members, and close friends may provide valuable insight regarding psychological and social status and should be included in the screening process (and program) whenever possible.

Benefits

In examining the potential benefits of pulmonary rehabilitation, one should consider the effects of the individual program components as well as more general outcomes common to all programs. The typical multidisciplinary, comprehensive pulmonary rehabilitation program includes a variety of treatment modalities that may be individualized according to the needs of each patient and to the resources and expertise available in a particular program. In evaluating the benefits of pulmonary rehabilitation, therefore, it is often difficult to determine which of the many integrally related program components are most responsible for specific outcomes. For example, almost any specific treatment (e.g., education, exercise) provided by well-trained and enthusiastic personnel inevitably also will provide important elements of psychosocial support and motivation for these sick and disabled patients.

Another potential limitation of the available pulmonary rehabilitation literature is that many of the clinical studies have included small numbers of patients. Certain benefits, although dramatic in individuals, may not occur in all subjects; therefore, statistical analysis of group means may miss real benefits for some patients.[118]

In this section, the evidence for the more general outcomes and anticipated benefits that may result from participation in a pulmonary rehabilitation program will be examined first. Then, the evidence for expected changes from specific components will be discussed.

General Benefits

Hospitalizations/Medical Resources

Comprehensive pulmonary rehabilitation programs have been shown to be a cost-effective means of producing significant benefits for patients with COPD. Several studies have compared the number of hospital days and other medical resources used by patients before and after participation in a pulmonary rehabilitation program.[79] Given the high costs of acute care hospitalizations for these patients, the potential savings from a reduction in hospital days alone is significant.

Several studies have examined the hospitalization and cost savings within the first year after pulmonary rehabilitation. Many of these estimated costs are outdated and the potential savings are even greater today. Lertzman and Cherniack reported an average decrease of 20 hospital days per year from pulmonary rehabilitation, which resulted in an estimated savings of $2,000 per patient based on a Canadian hospital cost of $100 per day in 1976.[105] Petty et al. reported a 38% reduction in total hospital days (868 to 542) among 85 patients with COPD evaluated 1 year after entry to a pulmonary rehabilitation program compared with the year before entry.[138] In a randomized, controlled study, Jensen reported that pulmonary rehabilitation led to significantly fewer hospitalizations over 6 months of follow-up in patients with COPD with "high-risk" markers for psychosocial problems.[92] In an evaluation of an inpatient pulmonary rehabilitation program, Agle et al. reported 30 hospital admissions among 24 patients in the year before rehabilitation compared with only 5 admissions in the subsequent year.[2]

Several investigators have examined the long-term effects of pulmonary rehabilitation. Hudson et al. reported a considerable reduction in hospitalizations for pulmonary disease in 64 patients who participated in a comprehensive pulmonary rehabilitation program and who had undergone follow-up after 4 years (44 alive, 20 dead).[89] In the 44 patients alive 4 years after the program, the number of hospital days in the year before the program (529) was reduced by 73% in year 1 (145 days), 49% in year 2 (270 days), 47% in year 3 (278 days), and 61% in year 4 (207 days). This benefit was most striking in the 14 of the 44 patients who had been hospitalized in the year before the program, whose hospitalization days decreased from 38 to 10 days per patient comparing the year before vs the year after rehabilitation. Including the 20 patients who died, in the 64 patients there were 631 days of hospitalization in the year before the rehabilitation program vs 309 days (52% reduction) in the first year and 350 days (45% reduction) in the second year after the program.

The work of other investigators corroborates these findings. Johnson et al. reported a 55% decrease in hospital days in the year after vs the year before an inpatient pulmonary rehabilitation program in 96 patients with severe COPD (mean FEV_1 = 0.87 L).[93] There was an average decrease of 23 hospital days per year in these patients. This group has also reported a cost-benefit analysis of long-term follow-up of 193 patients who underwent inpatient pulmonary rehabilitation.[110] They estimated an average reduction of 21 hospital days per surviving patient per year. Despite the cost of inpatient rehabilitation ($9,000 in 1982), they estimated a net cost saving of $11,200 per patient over 2.8 years of follow-up due to reduced hospitalizations.

Hodgkin et al. have reported an average reduction from 19 hospital days in the year before rehabilitation to nearly 6 days in the first year after the program in 80 patients with COPD. Estimating the cost of a hospital day at $400 at that time, the savings from reduced hospitalization alone amount to $416,000 for the group, or $5,200 per patient in the first year.[128] In addition, their improvement was maintained for the 8 years of follow-up for which data were analyzed. The benefit was seen both in survivors and nonsurvivors over the period of follow-up.[79,80,84]

Sneider et al. analyzed hospital cost data for 5 years before and after rehabilitation for 50 patients randomly selected from each of three groups: (1) those interviewed but not enrolling in rehabilitation; (2) those who received education but not exercising; and (3) those who completed all phases of the program.[163] They found that the group that completed the full program had a decrease of 1.8 hospital days per year per patient (compared from the baseline of 7.2 days per year). At 1987 prices, this represented a cost savings of $2,147 per patient. In contrast, patients in the interviewed-only group had an increase of 3.2 hospital days per year and those in the education-only group had an increase of 2.1 days per year.

Improvement in the overall level of care for patients with COPD from pulmonary rehabilitation has also been suggested. In a study comparing 252 patients with COPD who participated in a comprehensive pulmonary rehabilitation program with 50 nonrehabilitation patients selected from an outpatient clinic, Haas and Cardon reported that, after 5 years, 8% of the rehabilitated patients and 17% of controls were placed in a nursing home. In addition, 19% of the rehabilitation group vs only 5% of controls were able to provide their own self-care at that time.[74]

Quality of Life/Symptoms

For patients, the major benefits of pulmonary rehabilitation are related to improvement in quality of life, reduction in debilitating respiratory symptoms, increase in exercise tolerance and level of physical activity, more independence and ability to perform activities of daily living, and improvement in psychological function with less anxiety and depression and increased feelings of hope, control, and self-esteem.[138] Therefore, to evaluate the effectiveness of pulmonary rehabilitation, it is important to incorporate measurements that reflect changes in "quality of life." Several investigators have developed and validated such instruments for use in patients with chronic lung diseases.[11,95,96,140]

The success of pulmonary rehabilitation in reducing health care use in patients with COPD may be closely related to the improvement in quality of life and patient symptoms. As pointed out by Traver, health care use by patients with COPD is dependent on important factors other than just the severity of underlying lung disease.[179] She reported that patients with "high" vs "low" use of emergent health care resources had similar spirometric indices of lung function but significantly greater impairment in quality of life and more symptoms, including irritability, anxiety, helplessness, nervousness, and alienation. Therefore, changes in both respiratory and psychosocial symptom complexes are important in understanding the potential benefits of pulmonary rehabilitation.

Bebout et al. administered a quality of life questionnaire to 75 patients with COPD an average of 92 months (minimum of 24 months) after a comprehensive rehabilitation program.[17] Among the 43 patients who responded at follow-up, greater than 50% reported improvement in their dyspnea classification, ability to go outside, frequency of difficult breathing episodes, and self-assurance.

In a long-term study of multidisciplinary pulmonary rehabilitation in 31 consecutive patients, Guyatt et al. included measures of quality of life using the chronic respiratory disease questionnaire.[73]

Twenty-four patients demonstrated improvement in quality of life measured 2 weeks after completing the rehabilitation program. Over 6 months of follow-up, the improved quality of life was sustained in 11 of these 24 patients.

In a report of the results of an outpatient pulmonary rehabilitation program in 197 patients in a community hospital, Mall and Medeiros reported that 77% of patients with worse than class 1 dyspnea improved their dyspnea classification.[111]

In a randomized, controlled study of the influence of behavioral factors on the effectiveness of exercise in patients with COPD, Atkins et al. administered extensive psychosocial outcome parameters including an established Quality of Well-Being Scale.[11] After 3 months of exercise and behavioral intervention (without formal pulmonary rehabilitation) and an additional 3 months of follow-up, they found that compared to a no-treatment control group, 3 different experimental groups demonstrated significantly greater positive changes in the Quality of Well-Being measurements. Using these data to estimate and compare the cost-effectiveness of intervention strategies in producing a well-year of life, the investigators concluded that even this modest treatment program resulted in significant cost-benefits for these patients.

Improving patient symptoms and quality of life is certainly an important outcome of medical care. There are only a few experimental studies that have systematically examined quality of life changes from pulmonary rehabilitation. In clinical practice, however, both patients and physicians report considerable symptomatic benefits, which are a major factor contributing to the enthusiasm many of these individuals have for such programs. Further research studies in this area are needed and should incorporate established measures to examine the symptomatic changes reported by many patients.

Pulmonary Function Tests

Since most pulmonary rehabilitation programs admit patients when they are stable and already on appropriate standard medical treatment, pulmonary rehabilitation has not resulted in consistent improvement in tests of lung function in patients with COPD.[80,119,127,138,139]

In a randomized clinical trial of medical and rehabilitative therapy vs medical therapy alone, Ambrosino et al. reported a significant increase in FEV_1 and PaO_2 with a decrease in $PaCO_2$ in the experimental group only.[4] Similar but nonsignificant trends were seen in the control group. However, patients were enrolled in this study before any therapy, so these findings cannot be attributed to the rehabilitation components.

In a randomized trial of exercise training in 39 patients with COPD and coal workers pneumoconiosis, Cockcroft et al. found no change in FEV_1 in either trained or control subjects, whereas FVC increased slightly in both groups.[47]

In a controlled nonrandomized study of 33 patients with COPD, Sinclair and Ingram reported an increase in FVC only in the trained patients with no other changes in lung function in either group (including measures of FEV_1 and diffusion).[161]

In a randomized controlled study of exercise training in 28 patients with COPD, McGavin et al. reported no significant changes in spirometric indices in either the experimental or control group despite significant improvement in exercise performance noted in the trained patients.[112]

In an evaluation of 30 patients with COPD 1 year after participation in a pulmonary rehabilitation program, Fishman and Petty reported a significant improvement in maximal voluntary ventilation (and exercise tolerance) despite no change in $FEV_{1.0}$, PaO_2, or $PaCO_2$.[60]

In a study of exercise training in 21 patients with COPD compared with 8 control subjects, Chester et al. found no change in pulmonary function or in rest and exercise measurements of arterial blood gases or hemodynamics from right heart catheterization after training in either group despite improved work tolerance in the trained patients.[41] Similar results were observed by Alpert et al. in an extensive evaluation of 5 patients with COPD before and after 18 weeks of exercise training.[3]

Survival

It is clear that survival for patients with recognized COPD is reduced considerably to approximately 50% at 5 years and 25% at 10 years.[180] This poor rate of survival is related largely to the fact that the diseases are typically recognized and diagnosed at an advanced stage. Studies that have examined the survival of COPD patients after pulmonary rehabilitation have shown variable results.[79] To date, there are no published prospective, randomly controlled studies of pulmonary rehabilitation that have examined patient survival.

In a retrospective study of 75 patients with COPD and a mean follow-up of 92 months, Bebout et al. reported improved survival after a comprehensive pulmonary rehabilitation program compared with that reported in other published studies.[17] However, patients in this study had less severe disease than in the comparison studies. In patients with less severe disease (FEV_1 greater than 1.24 L), survival at 2 to 7 years was significantly greater than that reported in the literature for the natural history of COPD.

In an analysis of 11 years of experience with pulmonary rehabilitation, Sneider et al. compared survival in patients with COPD who completed the pulmonary rehabilitation program with other COPD patients seen in the same institution.[163] They found higher survival for the rehabilitation patients each year over 10 years of follow-up. Survival rates were similar to those reported by Bebout et al.,[17] even though these patients had more severe disease.

In a prospective study of 182 consecutive patients who participated in a comprehensive outpatient pulmonary rehabilitation program, Sahn et al. reported 41% survival at 5 years and 17% at 10 years.[155] However, this program was conducted in Denver at altitude, a factor that would reduce survival for patients with COPD. Comparing data at 2.5 years of follow-up with a study of the natural history of COPD for patients at comparable altitude,[144] survival was found to be significantly improved (67% vs 50%).

In a study comparing 252 rehabilitated patients with 50 control subjects selected from an outpatient clinic, Haas and Cardon reported 5-year mortality rates from respiratory failure of 22% in the rehabilitated patients and 42% in control subjects.[74]

Among 985 patients who participated in a clinical trial of intermittent positive pressure breathing, Anthonisen et al. reported a marked improvement in survival over 3 years of follow-up compared with other published studies in similar patient groups.[8] The authors concluded that this improved survival was due, at least in part, to the comprehensive assessment, education, care, and follow-up (similar to that provided in pulmonary rehabilitation).

Occupational Changes

Vocational rehabilitation may be difficult to achieve once the patient has become disabled from severe lung disease.[105] In addition, COPD typically presents in older patients who are more likely to be retired and less inclined to return to gainful employment. For the younger, working patient, the optimal time for rehabilitation, then, is before the patient becomes disabled. Patients with less severe

disease may be able to return to work and increase their performance of vocational and recreational activities. In addition to the level of pulmonary impairment, an individual's potential and success in vocational rehabilitation will depend on other factors including age, intelligence, motivation, education, capacity for retraining, physical demands of a particular job, and support and understanding from an employer.[54,97]

In an evaluation of 182 consecutive patients enrolled in a pulmonary rehabilitation program, Petty et al. found that 32% were working at least part time on entry to the program.[137] Compared with the nonworking patients, working patients were significantly younger and had better exercise tolerance despite the fact that there were no significant differences in measurements of pulmonary function or arterial blood gases. These observations emphasize the importance of variables other than the degree of pulmonary impairment per se in determining an individual's ability to maintain gainful employment.

In a separate report, among 85 patients with COPD evaluated 1 year after participation in a pulmonary rehabilitation program, Petty et al. reported that 21 patients were employed at least part-time during the whole year and 35 additional patients were employed during at least part of the year.[138] Also, 8 patients returned to work after more than 1 year of unemployment.

Haas and Cardon found that 25% of 252 patients with COPD who participated in a pulmonary rehabilitation program, which included vocational counseling and rehabilitation, were able to engage in full-time work 5 years after the program. In comparison, only 3% of 50 control patients selected from an outpatient clinic were able to work 5 years later. An additional 19% of the rehabilitation patients vs only 5% control subjects were able to care for themselves.[74]

In a controlled clinical trial, Lustig et al. randomly allocated 45 patients with COPD into three groups: (1) pulmonary rehabilitation; (2) psychotherapy alone; and (3) no treatment.[108] They found that, compared with the no-treatment group, patients in both the pulmonary rehabilitation and psychotherapy groups showed improvement in measurements of psychological function. However, although all patients were given vocational counseling, the group receiving pulmonary rehabilitation had significantly more patients subsequently engaged in vocational activities. Of the 15 patients in each group, there were 11 rehabilitation patients compared with only 4 psychotherapy and 3 no-treatment patients employed 6 weeks later.

Kass et al. reported on the work status of 147 patients followed-up at a mean of 31 months after admission to a pulmonary rehabilitation program.[97] They found that 21% were still working, 23% worked for at least 6 months but were not still working, 24% did not work after rehabilitation, and 32% had died. They found that physiological measurements (e.g., FEV_1) were more highly correlated with potential for vocational rehabilitation for these patients than measured psychologic factors, but observed that, for an individual patient, achieving successful vocational status is dependent on a number of variables. In a subsequent report, this group used results of the Minnesota Multiphasic Personality Inventory (MMPI) to predict vocational adjustment in these patients.[61] They found that patients who worked more than 6 months were more gregarious, self-confident, and more likely to use denial. In contrast, patients who did not work were more anxious, self-doubting, and irritable.

Long-Term Follow-Up

Few studies of pulmonary rehabilitation programs have systematically followed patients for more than a few months. In the short-term, patients frequently demonstrate dramatic improvements including reduced symptoms, increased tolerance for exercise and physical activities, and better quality of life. However, in some patients, beneficial effects appear to decrease over the longer term. Therefore, in evaluating and structuring pulmonary rehabilitation programs, it is important to consider longer term outcomes and to consider whether additional sessions for reinforcement and maintenance would be worthwhile in these programs.

Guyatt et al. followed 31 consecutive patients enrolled in a multidisciplinary inpatient pulmonary rehabilitation program for 6 months.[73] Primary outcome measures included a chronic respiratory disease questionnaire to measure quality of life and a 6-minute walk test to assess exercise tolerance. Of the 28 patients who completed the program, 21 were retested at 6 months. The 10 patients who were not tested at 6 months were evaluated by telephone interview (they had lower baseline health status than the 21 formally tested at 6 months). Results indicated that 24 patients demonstrated improvement in quality of life 2 weeks after

the rehabilitation program (77% of 31 patients enrolled, 86% of 28 patients who completed the program). After 6 months, however, improvement in quality of life was sustained in 11 patients but declined in 20 patients (35% vs 65% of 31 patients enrolled; 39% vs 71% of 28 patients completing the program). The 6-minute walk test was administered to 17 patients at 6 months of follow-up. In these 17 patients, the distance walked improved significantly at 2 weeks and declined somewhat over 6 months, but remained significantly greater than baseline measurement. Also of note is the finding that 13 of the 28 patients who completed the program stopped exercising within a month of discharge from the program. As in many other studies, spirometry measures of lung function did not change significantly after rehabilitation. However, this uncontrolled study does not allow evaluation of similar changes in patients not enrolling in a rehabilitation program and, therefore, subject to the natural history of disease.

In a randomized trial of exercise training in 39 patients, Cockcroft et al. reported a significant increase in the 12-minute walk distance in trained patients compared with controls at 2 months of follow-up.[47] Most of this improvement was maintained in the exercise patients for up to 7 months. However, the difference from controls was not significant at 4 months due to an increase in exercise performance in controls.

Fishman and Petty re-evaluated 30 patients with COPD 1 year after participation in a pulmonary rehabilitation program.[60] They found statistically significant improvement in maximal voluntary ventilation (without change in FEV_1), walking exercise tolerance, and patient ratings of affective distress. However, as the authors point out, it is difficult to assess the overall impact of the program without reference to a control, nontreatment group since many of the measured variables expected to worsen over one year "did not change."

Tydeman et al. enrolled 24 patients with COPD in a supervised exercise training program.[181] After patients reached maximum improvement with supervised training, they continued to exercise at home but were randomly allocated to continued weekly supervised sessions or no supervision. Sixteen patients completed the trial. The length of time to reach peak performance on the variety of exercise tasks used ranged from 26 to 51 weeks (mean, 36 weeks). For the 12-minute walk test, these patients demonstrated a 42% increase, most of which occurred over the first 4 weeks of training. On subsequent re-evaluation up to 6 months after the random allocation for follow-up, both groups of patients maintained the improvement in exercise performance with daily home walking regardless of whether they had regular supervision. These findings suggest that, for motivated patients who complete the training program and maintain home exercise, the benefits of exercise training can be maintained without frequent supervision.

Therefore, it is difficult to critically evaluate long-term outcomes of pulmonary rehabilitation programs or components without appropriate clinical trials, which control for the expected progression of disease and changes in function over time.

Specific Components

In evaluating the effectiveness of pulmonary rehabilitation, separating the individual components may be artificial and somewhat arbitrary. Nevertheless, it is important to try to gain some understanding of the rationale for incorporating specific treatment modalities into such programs. Therefore, in this section, the evidence for the effectiveness of program components most commonly included in pulmonary rehabilitation will be examined.

Education

Success of a pulmonary rehabilitation program is dependent on patients and family members being actively involved and improving their understanding of the COPD disease process and practical ways of coping with its debilitating symptoms. Therefore, education has been recommended and included as an integral part of comprehensive rehabilitation programs.[68,105] Studies that have examined the effects of the individual program components have shown that even patients with severe disease can learn to understand their disease better.[126] Standardized instruments to evaluate knowledge have been developed and validated.[87] However, it is less clear whether education alone can lead to improved health status for such patients. In addition to knowledge, most patients require specific, individual strategies for changing behavior along with encouragement, practice, and positive feedback. A variety of teaching formats have been used, but instruction needs to be tailored to each patient's learning ability (e.g., problems of older patients).

Several studies have evaluated the effects of education for patients with COPD. Howland et al. performed a controlled study of the effect of an education program on health status of patients with COPD in two matched communities.[88] In one community, patients with COPD were identified, assessed, and offered an education program. In the other community, patients were only identified, assessed, and notified of the findings. In the education intervention community, patients with more severe disease received six 2-hour sessions on lung disease and various strategies for treating and coping with it. Patients with mild disease received three 2-hour sessions emphasizing prevention of impairment. Classes were taught in small groups of 6 to 12 patients allowing for group discussion. Patients in both communities were evaluated with measures of functional health status, psychosocial variables, and health status with a locus of control instrument. Analysis was performed on 213 patients who completed the education program in the experimental community (41% of patients with COPD identified in that community) vs 325 patients who completed both evaluations in the control community (80% of patients with COPD identified). Results indicated that the health education program had no significant impact on any measure of health status including measures of symptom status, physical function, mental health, or social function. Only the health locus of control was significantly different after the intervention indicating that patients who received the education program were more likely to believe that they could control their own health. These findings suggest that, although education programs administered alone may improve patients' knowledge of disease, they may not produce significant change in patients' health status unless accompanied by other components typically included in comprehensive pulmonary rehabilitation programs.

In another study, Ashikaga et al. evaluated a community-based education program that included didactic material, demonstration of self-help skills, and group discussions dealing with psychosocial aspects of COPD.[10] Compared with control participants who received written material only, the program subjects demonstrated a significant improvement in their knowledge of COPD. However, the control subjects had significant improvements in their Perceived Chance of Improvement and in Social Disability. These short-term findings suggest that the generally positive information presented to controls, without counseling or open discussion, may have resulted in a false expectation of improvement. This emphasizes the importance of providing time for counseling patients in the proper interpretation of educational material presented.

Respiratory and Chest Physiotherapy

Many patients with COPD use, abuse, and are confused about respiratory and chest physiotherapy techniques. As part of a comprehensive rehabilitation program, each individual patient's needs and use of respiratory care techniques is assessed and instruction provided in proper use. Such evaluation and instruction may include chest physiotherapy techniques to enhance mucociliary clearance and control excess secretions; breathing training techniques to relieve and control dyspnea and improve ventilatory function; and proper use of respiratory care equipment including nebulizers, metered dose inhalers, and oxygen.[105,153] Although some remain skeptical about their efficacy, clear objective and subjective benefits have resulted from use of these techniques.[40]

Bronchial Hygiene.   Patients with chronic lung disease have abnormalities in lung clearance mechanisms, which make them more susceptible to problems with retained secretions and infections. Therefore, rehabilitation programs typically teach appropriate coughing and chest physiotherapy techniques for secretion control.[6,49] These are important for patients with excess mucous production during periods of exacerbation of disease and on a regular basis as preventive health care measures for patients with chronic sputum production. Studies have demonstrated that properly applied postural drainage with chest percussion or clapping increases the rate of removal of radioactive aerosol from the airways[16] and the volume of expectorated sputum in pulmonary patients with chronic excess bronchial secretions.[40] They are also as beneficial as bronchoscopy in clearing lobar atelectasis.[40] However, they have not been clearly shown to produce clinical improvement in the acute inhospital setting for patients with uncomplicated pneumonia[71] or with acute exacerbations of COPD.[9]

Several studies have reported benefits from the techniques taught, which typically include controlled coughing, postural drainage, and chest vibration and/or percussion.[100,120,131,142,153,168,169] The efficacy of the individual techniques is difficult to determine from the literature; available evidence suggests that postural drainage and controlled coughing (or the forced expiration technique)[141] may be the most effective components.[166,168] Administration of nebulized saline or bronchodilators may increase secretion clearance.[167] These techniques are most effective in patients with a large amount of sputum (e.g., >30 ml/day), whether from chronic or acute conditions. The benefits in patients without excess sputum is less clear; also, these techniques may induce bronchoconstriction in patients with reactive airways. Whether the chest physical therapy techniques add significantly to effective coughing alone is also not clear.

The use of mucolytic agents to reduce viscosity of secretions is of questionable benefit; in several studies, they do not appear to be any more effective than placebo.[131] However, one large multicenter, randomized, placebo-controlled clinical trial of mucolytic therapy reported an improvement in cough frequency, cough severity, chest discomfort, ease of raising sputum, and overall health status for patients treated with iodinated glycerol after 8 weeks of therapy.[135]

Finally, the use of intermittent positive pressure breathing (IPPB) has been evaluated systematically and found to be ineffective.[91,102]

Breathing Training Techniques.   Pulmonary rehabilitation programs frequently teach certain breathing training techniques aimed at helping patients to relieve and control breathlessness and to counteract physiological abnormalities related to chronic airflow obstruction (e.g., mechanical disadvantage of inspiratory muscles and increased respiratory work due to increased resting lung volume).[6,33,40,49,59,118,153] Such techniques may include diaphragmatic and pursed-lips breathing aimed at improving the ventilatory pattern (i.e., slow respiratory rate, increase tidal volume), preventing dynamic airway compression, improving respiratory synchrony of abdominal and thoracic musculature, and improving gas exchange.[120]

A review of clinical studies evaluating the effects of these breathing training techniques points out that improvement in clinical symptoms (e.g., dyspnea) is a more consistent finding than associated measurable changes in physiologic parameters. Also, as pointed out by Miller,[118] in evaluating these techniques it is difficult to separate the possible contributions of each of the various methods used since they are frequently taught together and integrated with other components such as patient education and psychosocial support.

The most consistent physiologic change observed after breathing training in patients with

COPD is an increase in tidal volume and a decrease in respiratory rate. Motley demonstrated improvement in gas exchange associated with controlled, slow deep breathing in 35 patients with COPD.[122] He noted an increase in arterial oxygen saturation in 33 patients associated with a decrease in $PaCO_2$ and a slight improvement in steady-state diffusing capacity with the controlled breathing technique.

Other studies have reported improvement in ventilatory efficiency with a technique of paced slow breathing.[134,158] However, this technique does not appear to be associated with the same degree of symptomatic relief commonly experienced with pursed-lip breathing.

Diaphragmatic Breathing. The diaphragmatic breathing technique was described by Barach[12,14] and Miller[118] as a maneuver in which the patient attempts to coordinate abdominal wall expansion with inspiration and to slow expiration through pursed lips.[59] The primary aim is to slow respiratory rate and increase tidal volume, which has been demonstrated in several studies along with improvement in patient symptoms.

Miller evaluated the effects of 6 to 8 weeks of diaphragmatic breathing training in a group of 24 patients with stable COPD.[117] He found a significant increase in diaphragmatic excursion (measured fluoroscopically from maximum expiration to maximum inspiration). This was associated with a significant increase (34%) in resting tidal volume and decrease (42%) in respiratory rate without change in total ventilation at rest or with exercise. This improved ventilatory efficiency resulted in improved gas exchange with increased arterial oxygen saturation, decreased arterial PCO_2, and increased exercise tolerance with less dyspnea. In addition, vital capacity and maximal breathing capacity increased 23% and 37%, respectively.

Sinclair studied the effects of diaphragmatic breathing accompanied by relaxation therapy over several weeks in 22 patients with COPD and found no change in measurements of pulmonary function but an increase in diaphragmatic excursion.[162] Fourteen of the patients, however, noted symptomatic improvement associated with the treatment program. Similar results were reported by Becklake et al., who noted that 8 of 10 patients reported subjective improvement associated with diaphragmatic breathing and relaxation therapy; however, there were no significant changes in measurements of pulmonary function.[18]

In a pilot study, Williams et al. examined spirometry, 12-minute walk distance, and ratings of perceived exertion in 8 patients with COPD after 3 weeks of placebo physiotherapy and 3 weeks of diaphragmatic breathing.[187] They found no change in any of the measured parameters over the course of the study.

Sackner et al. studied the effects of diaphragmatic breathing on distribution of ventilation in 11 patients with COPD.[154] They found no change in indices of distribution calculated from the nitrogen-washout curve or from xenon ventilation lung scans associated with diaphragmatic breathing.

Pursed-Lips Breathing. Pursed-lips breathing is the other breathing training technique typically taught along with diaphragmatic breathing.[12,59,118] Pursed-lips breathing in patients with COPD was observed by Laennec as early as 1830 and advocated as a physical exercise for these patients in the early part of the 20th century.[13] It takes advantage of a maneuver often assumed naturally by some patients, in which the lips are used to narrow the airway during expiration. The aims are to slow the expiratory phase and to maintain positive pressure in the airways to "keep the airways open" and improve ventilatory efficiency, although these effects have not been clearly demonstrated.

Mueller et al. found that pursed-lips breathing led to an increase in tidal volume and decrease in respiratory rate in patients with COPD at rest and during exercise.[123] This led to an improvement in ventilatory efficiency, i.e., a decrease in the minute ventilation (V_E) needed for a given level of oxygen consumption (VO_2) (decrease in V_E/VO_2). Seven of 12 patients also experienced associated symptomatic relief of dyspnea.

Thoman et al. studied pursed-lips breathing in 21 patients with COPD and reported improved ventilation to poorly ventilated areas of the lung compared with normal breathing.[174] In addition, both pursed-lips and controlled rate breathing produced a significant change in the respiratory pattern with an increase in tidal volume and decrease in respiratory rate in each of 7 patients studied.

Tiep et al. compared pursed-lips breathing with general relaxation in 12 patients with COPD.[176] During pursed-lips breathing, patients were allowed to watch the digital readout of an ear oximeter. They found a significantly higher arterial oxygen saturation and tidal volume and lower respiratory rate during pursed-lips breathing. There was no change in minute ventilation.

Oxygen. Supplemental oxygen therapy has been shown to be beneficial for patients with significant resting arterial hypoxemia either from acute or chronic causes of lung disease.[23,24,66] Possible benefits of supplemental oxygen for nonhypoxemic patients or for patients with hypoxemia only under certain conditions (e.g., exercise, sleep) are less clearly defined.[7,22,26]

The effects on exercise tolerance of oxygen administered routinely to patients with COPD have demonstrated variable results. In a study of patients with COPD participating in a pulmonary rehabilitation program, Longo et al. found no significant improvement in breathlessness or exercise tolerance from oxygen administered at 2 or 4 L per minute compared with compressed air in 27 patients with COPD.[107] There was slight improvement, however, in the subset of patients with exercise-induced hypoxemia. On the other hand, Vyas et al. reported a significant increase in maximum work rate and oxygen uptake in 12 patients with COPD breathing 40% oxygen compared with room air administered in a double-blind fashion.[184] Zack and Palange reported a 28% increase in maximum exercise workload for patients with COPD entering a pulmonary rehabilitation program breathing oxygen at 4 L per minute compared with room air.[192] Davidson et al. found an improvement in rated dyspnea, endurance walking time, and 6-minute walking distance with 4 L per minute of oxygen independent of the degree of hypoxemia present at rest or with exercise.[55] In addition, the benefit from supplemental oxygen was not cancelled by the effort required to carry a portable oxygen cylinder. Bradley et al. compared maximum and endurance exercise performance on room air, compressed air, and supplemental oxygen at 5 L per minute in 26 patients with COPD.[27] They reported improvement in exercise endurance but not maximum work rate on supplemental oxygen compared to either room air or compressed air. Thus, it appears that supplemental oxygen administered routinely to patients with COPD may result in improvement in exercise endurance but variable changes in maximal exercise tolerance. The improvements may depend on the amount of oxygen administered.

Long-term, continuous oxygen therapy has been clearly shown to improve survival and reduce morbidity of hypoxemic patients with COPD.[6,7,114,129] In fact, at this time, this is the only treatment that has been proven to prolong survival in patients with severe COPD. Although continuous, ambulatory oxygen therapy for hypoxemic patients is feasible and safe, maintaining such patients on oxygen presents a number of problems.[66,136,175] These problems are particularly difficult for the more physically disabled and older patients who may need assistance in handling, using, and caring safely for such equipment.

Several new developments in this area have improved the efficiency of gas delivery and patient compliance with continuous therapy.[177] Using liquid oxygen as a gas source provides more oxygen for less weight in portable systems. Also, the use of transtracheal oxygen increases the efficiency of gas delivery to the patient (reducing oxygen flow requirement and prolonging duration of portable sources), improves patient compliance and avoids problems with nasal catheters.[44] However, patients need careful instruction in caring for and maintaining the catheter. The presence of another person (e.g., spouse) is particularly helpful in the daily care and replacement of the catheters. These problems are particularly important in older patients who should be screened carefully before implementing the procedure.

Psychosocial Support

An essential component of a comprehensive pulmonary rehabilitation program is psychosocial support.[6,105] From the realization that their disease is chronic and incurable, patients with COPD develop a variety of psychosocial symptoms reflecting their progressive feelings of hopelessness and inability to cope with their disease.[1,57,58,69,113,140,157,188] Depression is common.[106,113] Patients may show symptoms of anxiety (particularly fear of dyspnea), denial, anger, and isolation and become sedentary and dependent on family members, friends, and providers of medical services for their needs. They become overly concerned with other physical problems and psychosomatic symptoms. Sexual dysfunction and fear of sexual activities are common, often unspoken, consequences of chronic lung disease; patients can be helped by appropriate counseling from knowledgeable and supportive staff.[52,63,178] Patients with COPD have evidence of cognitive and neuropsychological dysfunction, possibly related to or exacerbated by the effects of hypoxemia on the brain. It has been demonstrated that a patient's psychological status is an important determinant of the respiratory symptoms reported.[53]

Successful pulmonary rehabilitation programs not only attend to physical problems but also to psychosocial ones. This is provided best by enthusiastic and supportive staff who are able to communicate effectively with patients and devote the time and effort necessary to understand and motivate them. Effective care of patients with COPD needs to pay attention to individual needs, which requires significant staff time with each patient.[69] Important family members and friends should be included in program activities so that they can understand and cope better with the patient's disease. Support groups and group therapy sessions are very effective. Patients with severe psychological disorders may benefit from individual counseling and psychotherapy. Psychotropic drugs generally should be reserved for patients with severe levels of psychological dysfunction.[69]

Several studies have reported significant relationships between psychosocial variables and outcome in treatment of patients with COPD. These highlight the importance of appropriate attention to psychosocial components in comprehensive care programs for these patients. Williams has reviewed many of the methodological problems in the psychosocial literature for chronic respiratory illness and emphasizes the importance of developing and using better objective instruments for studies evaluating the impact of COPD and proposed treatments on patients' lives and on society.[188]

In a randomized controlled trial of exercise training in 39 patients with COPD and coal workers pneumoconiosis, Cockcroft et al. found significant improvement in two tests administered to evaluate psychological variables in both the experimental and control groups.[46] These findings emphasize the problems in separating the effects of various components of a comprehensive pulmonary rehabilitation program, since patients may show improvement in psychological variables with even minimal attention and intervention such as participating in a clinical study as a control subject.

Jensen performed measurements of stress and social support in 59 patients with COPD and randomly assigned 30 "high-risk" patients to either a pulmonary rehabilitation, self-help support, or control group. He found that "high-risk" controls with high stress and low social support were hsopitalized significantly more frequently than either "low-risk" patients or the "high-risk" patients in the rehabilitation or self-help groups.[92] These findings emphasize the important influence of psychosocial status on hospitalization rates in

these patients and the beneficial effect of rehabilitation services in reducing their frequency.

Agle et al. evaluated physiologic and psychologic status in 24 patients before and after participation in a comprehensive inpatient pulmonary rehabilitation program.[2] They found that success in rehabilitation was correlated with the psychologic and not the physiologic measurements. Specifically, good responders tended to have less severe psychologic symptoms (depression, anxiety, body preoccupation) initially and to show improvement at 1 year. In particular, positive changes were related to desensitization to the fear of dyspnea and to increased patient autonomy in the control of symptoms. In contrast, poor responders had more psychologic dysfunction initially and showed little change after the program.

Relaxation Training. Because the dyspnea associated with chronic lung disease is closely associated with accompanying fear and anxiety, techniques of relaxation training have been incorporated into pulmonary rehabilitation programs. Techniques such as progressive relaxation, autogenic training, hypnosis, yoga, and transcendental meditation have been used in a variety of stress-related conditions and shown to be beneficial.[159] Since most relaxation techniques emphasize slow, rhythmic breathing, they may be particularly beneficial for patients with chronic lung diseases. Several studies have been conducted evaluating biofeedback and other relaxation type methods for patients with bronchial asthma[159]; however, there have been few studies specifically in patients with COPD.

Renfoe evaluated progressive muscle relaxation training in 10 patients with COPD compared with a control group, which was instructed to relax but not given specific instructions.[143] In this technique, patients are instructed to sequentially tense and then relax 16 different muscle groups. After the relaxation sessions, the experimental group demonstrated a significantly greater reduction in measurements of dyspnea and anxiety than the control subjects. Also, the change in dyspnea was significantly correlated with change in anxiety. These findings suggest that relaxation training can produce significant improvement in symptoms of both dyspnea and anxiety in these patients.

Other forms of therapy have also been used to help patients gain control of breathlessness and anxiety. Tandon compared yoga with standard physiotherapy, which included breathing training techniques in a randomized clinical trial in 24 patients with COPD.[170] Patients were not given any specific exercise training. After 9 months, the yoga patients demonstrated a significant increase in maximum work rate on a cycle ergometer not seen in the physiotherapy group. Also, a significantly greater number of the yoga patients reported improved exercise tolerance, quicker recovery after exertion, greater self-control over breathlessness, and improvement in their overall chest condition. Although yoga has not been used extensively in pulmonary patients, this study does indicate the possible benefits of such a technique provided by a practitioner experienced in helping patients to gain control over their symptoms.

Exercise

Exercise is generally considered to be an important component of pulmonary rehabilitation programs.[5,19,78,105,160] Reviews of the available evidence on the possible benefits of exercise reconditioning in patients with COPD have concluded that accepted benefits include increase in endurance, maximum oxygen consumption, and skill in task performance.[90,160] However, the optimal methods of training and the mechanisms of improvements seen have not yet been clearly defined in pulmonary patients.[22]

Of all the components provided in a pulmonary rehabilitation program, exercise is probably the most difficult in terms of personnel, equipment, and expertise. Principles derived in normal subjects or cardiac patients cannot be generalized to patients with chronic lung disease because of the different limitations to exercise performance and principles and problems of training.[20,22,28,35,121] Nevertheless, exercise reconditioning should be considered for all patients.

A variety of approaches have been used in exercise training for the patient with chronic lung disease. To be successful, the program should be tailored to the individual patient's physical abilities, interests, resources, and environment. For general application, techniques should be simple and inexpensive.[131] As in healthy individuals and other patient populations, benefits from exercise training are largely specific to the muscles and tasks involved in training. Patients tend to do best on activities and exercises for which they were trained.[130]

There is considerable evidence demonstrating both physiologic and psychologic improvements with exercise training in patients with chronic lung disease.[6,22,49,90] Patients may increase their maximum capacity and/or endurance for exercise and physical activity even though lung function does not usually change. Exercise training also provides an ideal opportunity for patients to learn their capacity for physical work and to use and practice methods for controlling dyspnea (e.g., breathing and relaxation techniques).

The exercise program needs to be safe and appropriate for each patient's interest, environment, and level of function. It should be based on the results of initial exercise testing. Training should use methods easily adapted to the home setting. Walking programs are particularly useful for physically limited patients. They have the added benefit of encouraging patients to expand their social horizons. In inclement weather, patients can frequently walk indoors (e.g., shopping malls). Other types of exercise (e.g., cycling, swimming) are also effective. Patients should be encouraged to incorporate regular exercise into activities they enjoy (e.g., golf, gardening). Since many patients with COPD have limited exercise tolerance, emphasis during training should be placed on increasing endurance. This will allow patients to become more functional within their physical limits. Increase in exercise level is also frequently possible as patients gain experience and confidence with their exercise program.

Benefits—Controlled Studies.   Since it is difficult to separate the effects of different possible program components in pulmonary rehabilitation, the benefits of exercise training are best evaluated in studies that attempt to control for the other components. Several controlled clinical trials of exercise training have been performed in this area.

Cockcroft et al. randomly assigned 39 male patients with both COPD and coal workers pneumoconiosis to a 6-week exercise training program (19 patients) or to a no-treatment control group (20 patients).[47] The exercise program included gymnasium activities on cycle ergometers and rowing machines, swimming, and walking. After the program, patients were instructed to continue walking and stair climbing exercises at home. The control group received no exercise advice, but after 4 months, they were allowed to enter the 6-week exercise program. In the 34 patients who completed the study (18 treatment, 16 control), patients in the exercise group experienced subjective benefits with decrease in reported symptoms and increased the 12-minute walk distance by 23% ($p<0.05$) after 2 months. Patients in the control group reported little change in subjective symptoms and increased their 12-minute walk distance by only 8% ($p=$NS). After 4 months, the 12-minute walk distance was not significantly different between groups, primarily because of continued improvement in control subjects. The treatment group maintained most of their improvement after 7 months of follow-up. For patients in the control group who began the exercise program after 4 months, there was a further significant increase in the 12-minute walk distance after training. FEV_1 did not change in either group during the study, whereas FVC increased slightly in both groups. Patients in this study also completed two questionnaires administered to assess psychologic variables.[46] Of note, both groups showed significant improvement in these psychologic tests, which were not significantly different between groups (although changes in the exercise group were slightly greater). The changes in the psychological tests were not correlated with changes in the 12-minute walk distance. These findings suggest that improvement in exercise tolerance was not related solely to changes in psychologic factors but also point out that even participating in a study with added attention may improve the psychological state of patients with COPD.

McGavin et al. randomly allocated 28 patients with COPD to a 3-month unsupervised stair-climbing home exercise program or to a nonexercise control group.[112] Four exercise patients did not complete the study (two for noncompliance, one death, one illness) leaving 12 in each group. Significantly more patients in the exercise group noted subjective improvement in sense of well-being, breathlessness, cough, and sputum. There was also a significant increase in exercise performance in the trained patients vs controls. The 12-minute walk distance increased 6% in the exercise group and decreased 2% in control subjects. The improvement in exercise patients was accompanied by a significant increase in stride length, indicating improvement in mechanical efficiency of walking. On the maximal cycle ergometer test, maximum work load increased 23% in the exercise group ($p<0.05$) vs a 4% decrease in control subjects ($p=$ NS) whereas $\dot{V}O_2$max increased 16% ($p=$

NS) in trained patients vs a 12% decrease in control subjects ($p<0.05$).

Sinclair and Ingram assigned 17 patients with COPD who lived within their city to an exercise training program and used 16 patients who lived outside the city as a nonexercise control group.[161] Exercise training consisted of a daily 12-minute walking distance test and supervised stair climbing exercise. Training was begun in the hospital and continued at home with weekly supervision. Patients were followed for up to 12 months. The exercise group demonstrated improvement in the 12-minute walk distance, which was maintained at 12 months, and subjective improvements in well-being, dyspnea, and daily activities. The nonequivalent control group did not show these changes. Improvement in exercise performance in the trained patients was associated with a decrease in the number of steps and increase in stride length, indicating improvement in the mechanical efficiency of walking.

Ambrosino et al. randomly assigned 23 patients to a medical and rehabilitative therapy group and 28 patients to medical therapy alone for 1 month.[4] Rehabilitative therapy included breathing control techniques of relaxation and slow breathing, diaphragmatic breathing, and pursed-lip breathing. Patients were not given specific exercise training. The authors reported improvement in maximal exercise tolerance on a cycle ergometer in the experimental group. In addition, these patients demonstrated improved efficiency of their ventilatory pattern with a decrease in respiratory rate and increase in tidal volume. These changes were not present in the control group.

Busch and McClements randomly allocated 20 patients with advanced COPD to a home-based exercise program or to a control group whose members were visited by a physical therapist but not instructed in exercise.[32] After 18 weeks, they found a significant difference between groups in physical work capacity on an incremental cycle ergometer test; this difference was due to a 3% increase in the exercise group vs a 28% decrease in the control group. These differences were not present in a home exercise test performed at 6-week intervals or in symptom scores of dyspnea. However, for analysis, the authors excluded three patients in the exercise group who were noncompliant with training and three patients in the control group—one who died and two who began exercising on their own. In the remaining patients, the exercise group appeared to have lower baseline exercise tolerance. This exclusion allows analysis of the effects of exercise training, but highlights the problems of trying to separate individual components of a rehabilitation program when patients may change behavior due to other interventions (e.g., begin exercising after enrolling in the study and being visited by a physical therapist). Nevertheless, these results emphasize the importance of a control group in such studies because "treated" patients with COPD who change little over time may, in fact, be significantly better than "untreated" patients whose function often declines.

Booker randomly allocated 128 patients with COPD to one of three groups: control, exercise, or physiotherapy (exercise plus breathing control techniques).[25] Over 12 months of follow-up, patients in both experimental groups demonstrated significant improvement in measures on a daily activities questionnaire and less mood disturbance. There was no statistically significant change in the 6-minute walk distance in any of the three groups. However, Booker points out the possible limitation of using a timed walking test to evaluate results of such programs, since patients with COPD are typically taught to take a longer time with activities to achieve more with less distress. These changes would not be reflected in a timed exercise test, which measures maximum distance covered in a set time.

Strijbos et al. studied 30 patients with COPD randomly assigned to either home care rehabilitation (reconditioning, relaxation, and breathing exercises) or control groups.[165] After 12 weeks of twice-weekly 30-minute sessions, patients in the rehabilitation group demonstrated significant improvement in maximum exercise tolerance and symptom ratings of perceived dyspnea and muscle fatigue. There were no changes in the control group patients.

Chester et al. compared the effects of exercise training in 21 patients with COPD with 8 control subjects who were not randomly selected.[41] The trained patients demonstrated significant improvement in total treadmill work associated with a decrease in oxygen consumption and minute ventilation at comparable levels of work. Control subjects showed no increase in work tolerance. There were no changes in either group in resting pulmonary function or rest and exercise measures of gas exchange and hemodynamics. The authors concluded that the improved work tolerance was

related importantly to improved efficiency of walking and desensitization to the sensation of dyspnea.

Benefits—Uncontrolled Studies. There are numerous reports from uncontrolled studies that demonstrate improved exercise performance after exercise training in patients with COPD performed either alone or as part of a more formal pulmonary rehabilitation program (e.g., summary Table 4 in report of Holle et al.).[86] In this section, several of these studies will be highlighted.

In one of the earlier studies, Pierce et al. reported on the results of treadmill exercise training over 3 to 16 weeks in 9 patients with severe COPD (mean FEV_1 = 0.93 L).[139] All patients studied demonstrated improved exercise endurance and maximum tolerance with an increase in maximal treadmill speed (mean of 3.5 to 5.5 mph) and $\dot{V}O_2max$ (23% increase). In addition, the patients showed improved mechanical efficiency of work with a decrease in VO_2, heart rate, and V_E and a more rapid recovery after exercise. Similar results were reported by Paez et al. after 3 weeks of treadmill exercise training in 8 patients with COPD.[130] They found an increase in maximal treadmill speed (mean increase of 1.4 to 2.4 mph) and improved mechanical efficiency associated with a longer stride length during walking. $\dot{V}O_2max$ was not measured.

Vyas et al. trained 14 patients with COPD (mean FEV_1 = 0.92 L) daily on a cycle ergometer for an average of 10 weeks (range, 6 to 26 weeks).[183] For the 11 patients who completed the training program, there was a significant increase in maximal work rate (mean = +24%) and in $\dot{V}O_2max$ (mean = +10%, range of −5 to +35%). In contrast to the previous treadmill training studies, there was no change in mechanical efficiency on the cycle ergometer (i.e., no reduction in VO_2 at constant work rates).

Carter et al. reported results of short-term, high-intensity exercise training in 59 patients with COPD during an 11-day inpatient rehabilitation program.[34] The patients performed twice daily exercise on treadmills and cycle ergometers and were instructed to exercise near their ventilatory limits for 30 to 40 minutes per session with rests allowed, if necessary. Results indicated increases in peak work level on a cycle ergometer, oxygen uptake, and ventilation after the program despite minimal changes in pulmonary function. The improvements were maintained at 3 months follow-up. These findings suggest that the increase in maximum work tolerance was related to improvements in maximum sustained ventilation and ventilatory efficiency, since the increase in peak exercise ventilation was due primarily to an increase in tidal volume.

Holle et al. reported results of a 6-week exercise program with an initial target set at 80% of peak work load.[86] In 44 patients who completed the training and follow-up testing, they found a 73% increase in peak METS estimated from treadmill work levels (3.28 to 5.46) whereas measured $\dot{V}O_2$max increased only 15% from 1.02 to 1.11 L/min. FEV_1, HRmax, and $V_E$max did not change. These findings suggest significant changes in mechanical efficiency of walking as a primary mechanism of the improvement in exercise performance. Also, in 24 patients who returned for follow-up testing at 12 ± 3 months, 89% of the peak exercise performance was maintained.

Mall and Medeiros reported the results of an outpatient pulmonary rehabilitation program in a community hospital in 197 patients.[111] After 6 weeks of exercise training, they found an increase in maximal work load on incremental treadmill testing accompanied by lower heart rate and respiratory rate. However, $\dot{V}O_2$max did not change, indicating that the change in work load was probably related to improvement in mechanical efficiency of walking.

Zack and Palange trained 63 patients with COPD in an outpatient pulmonary rehabilitation program in a community hospital at levels titrated to patient symptom tolerance.[192] Exercise training included walking and inspiratory muscle exercise. Among the 53 patients who completed the 12-week program, there was no significant increase in maximum exercise workload or $\dot{V}O_2$max on a cycle ergometer but a 51% increase in the 12-minute walk distance and a 57% increase in endurance time. However, with supplemental oxygen, there was a 14% increase in maximum cycle ergometer workload, 72% increase in 12-minute walk distance, and 98% increase in endurance time. These improvements were seen both in patients with and without exercise-induced hypoxemia and may have been related to reduction in the ventilatory requirement on oxygen.

Mohsenifar et al. evaluated 15 patients with COPD before and after participation in a 6-week pulmonary rehabilitation program.[119] They found little change in standard measurements of lung function or gas exchange. All patients reported a subjective improvement in exercise tolerance and demonstrated a significant increase in exercise endurance time which at least doubled in each patient. However, maximum work rate on a cycle ergometer did not change. The only measurable changes were a decrease in heart rate and blood lactate at comparable levels of exercise.

Woolf and Suero reported on the results of an inpatient exercise program for 14 patients with COPD.[191] They found improved exercise tolerance associated with a change in breathing pattern toward slower and deeper breathing. Also, after training there was a consistent decrease in blood lactate concentration.

Alpert et al. reported improved exercise tolerance in 5 patients after 18 weeks of exercise training associated with no change in measurements of pulmonary function, gas exchange, or hemodynamics from right heart catheterization.[3] They concluded that the increased exercise tolerance was probably due to improved muscle efficiency.

Tydeman et al. enrolled 24 patients with COPD in a supervised exercise training program.[181] In the 16 patients who were able to complete the training and study evaluations, they reported a 42% increase in 12-minute walk distance. There was a 22% increase in the first 4 weeks and further increase with continued training (mean time to maximum improvement of 36 weeks).

Christie reported on the results of stepping and walking exercise training in 11 patients with COPD and found that maximum work tolerance increased significantly in 9 of the 10 patients who completed the study (one patient died from unrelated causes).[43] This was also associated with an increase in $\dot{V}O_2$max and $V_E$max and decrease in V_E at submaximal work levels despite no significant change in lung function.

Bass et al. enrolled 12 patients with COPD in a cycle ergometry exercise training program over 18 weeks.[15] They found a significant increase in maximum work load in all 11 patients who completed the training program (one dropped out due to recurrent episodes of pneumonia). These patients also reported increased improvement in their activities of daily living associated with less breathlessness.

Most studies have reported results of short term exercise training in patients with COPD. However, there are several reports of longer terms results.

Nicholas et al. reported on the effects of 6 months of exercise training after a 3-month control period in 8 patients with COPD who completed the full study protocol (7 additional patients dropped out or were unable to complete the study).[127] They found an increase in exercise tolerance without change in ventilatory function or gas exchange measurements. They noted improvement in mechanical efficiency of walking as patients demonstrated improved mechanical work tolerance without concomitant changes in measured oxygen uptake. They also found that the patients tended to show improved exercise performance during the 3-month "control" period, suggesting that such patients may show improvements related to participation in a study with repeated exercise testing that is not necessarily related to the exercise training.

Brundin enrolled 31 patients with severe COPD (17 with and 14 without periods of respiratory failure) in a long-term study of cycle ergometry exercise training (accompanied by breathing exercises and chest physiotherapy).[29] Twenty-four patients were able to perform the training over the 6 to 18 months of follow-up. These patients noted subjective improvement in activity level with less dyspnea and demonstrated increased exercise tolerance.

Mertens et al. followed 13 patients with COPD during 1 year of exercise training and 6 patients for a second year.[115] They found an increase in predicted $\dot{V}O_2max$ (mean increase = 12%) at 1 year and noted that the magnitude of improvement was greater in those patients who were more compliant with their training regimen.

Exercise Prescription. An exercise prescription typically has four basic components: type of exercise, intensity, duration, and frequency. Although principles for prescribing exercise have been well established for healthy individuals or other patients (e.g., cardiac patients), the same cannot be said for the pulmonary patient. For the patient with advanced COPD, exercise tolerance is typically limited by maximum ventilation and the perception of breathlessness (dyspnea). Such patients frequently do not reach limits of cardiac or peripheral muscle performance seen in individuals without lung disease.

There has been much controversy about the selection of appropriate intensity targets for training patients with chronic lung disease.[78] For instance, in healthy individuals or cardiac patients, intensity is generally selected as a submaximal percentage of maximum heart rate or $\dot{V}O_2max$. Use of a target heart rate for pulmonary patients has been advocated by some authors,[78,80] although it is recognized that such targets may not be reliable for patients with more severe disease and others cast doubt on its usefulness.[19] One preliminary study has found that use of Karvonen's formula with 0.6 of the heart rate range [peak heart rate (PHR) minus resting heart rate (RHR)] produces an appropriate target heart rate (THR) for many patients with COPD; i.e., THR = [0.6 × (PHR − RHR)] + RHR.[83] Patients in this study were able to significantly increase the distance walked on 12-minute walk tests using this approach to exercise training.

However, it has also been reported that many patients with chronic lung disease, particularly when severe, can be trained at high percentages of maximum exercise tolerance that may approach or even exceed the maximum level reached on the initial maximum exercise test.[148] Patients with more mild disease can be trained at submaximal levels which are higher than the usual 60% to 70% of maximum expected in normals or cardiac patients. Therefore, some pulmonary rehabilitation programs tend to define exercise targets and progression during training by symptom tolerance rather than by strict heart rate or fixed work levels.[19,192] Ratings of perceived symptoms (e.g., breathlessness) help in teaching patients to exercise to "target" levels of breathing discomfort.[26] Therefore, after the initial exercise test to assess a patient's maximal exercise tolerance, a typical approach would be to begin training at a level that the patient can sustain with reasonable comfort for several minutes. This is an adequate starting point for training that emphasizes increasing endurance as well as level. Increase in time or level of exercise may then be made according to patient symptom tolerance.

In a study of intensive, inpatient exercise training in 59 patients with moderate to severe COPD, Carter et al. trained patients at levels near their ventilatory limits.[34] At baseline, after training, and 3 months later, they reported mean peak exercise ventilation of 94% to 100% of measured MVV. Patients improved maximum exercise levels and ventilation with training. These findings suggest that even patients with advanced disease can be trained successfully at maximal exercise levels.

Studies by Wasserman et al. suggest that determination of the anaerobic threshold (metabolic acidosis) during exercise may be helpful in selecting patients who might benefit most from exercise training. In one study, 14 of 22 patients with COPD showed evidence of a significant metabolic acidosis during exercise testing (often at a high percentage of $\dot{V}O_2$max.[185] The authors suggest that, in these patients at least, training at levels above the anaerobic threshold will lead to a reduced ventilatory requirement during exercise and, therefore, improved maximum exercise tolerance.[36]

Exercise-Induced Hypoxemia. A major problem in planning a safe exercise program for patients with COPD is the potential occurrence of exercise-induced hypoxemia. Patients who may or may not be hypoxemic at rest develop changes in arterial oxygenation that cannot be predicted reliably from resting measurements of pulmonary function or gas exchange.[151] Healthy individuals do not develop hypoxemia with exercise. Patients with mild COPD may demonstrate no change or an improvement in PaO_2 during exercise. However, PaO_2 with exercise in patients with moderate to severe COPD may increase, decrease, or not change. Therefore, it is important to measure arterial blood gases at rest and during exercise to detect significant exercise-induced hypoxemia and to decide how much oxygen is necessary for safe training. With the availability of convenient, portable systems for ambulatory oxygen delivery, hypoxemia is not a contraindication to exercise training.

Other Types of Exercise Training.

Upper Extremity. Exercise programs for patients with COPD have typically emphasized lower extremity training (e.g., walking, cycling). Other types of exercise may also be beneficial for the many physically limited pulmonary patients who have difficulty performing even simple activities of daily living. For instance, many patients with COPD report disabling dyspnea for daily activities involving the upper extremities (e.g., lifting, grooming) at work levels much lower than for the lower extremities.[38,149,171] Upper extremity exercise is accompanied by a higher ventilatory demand for a given level of work than for lower extremity exercise.[145,182] Also, because exercise training is generally specific to the muscles and tasks involved in training,[56,67,109,156,164] upper extremity exercises may be important in producing task specific benefits for pulmonary patients.[149]

Ries et al. evaluated two upper extremity home training programs in 45 patients with COPD participating concurrently in a multidisciplinary pulmonary rehabilitation program.[149] Compared with control subjects, who did not perform upper extremity training, patients in both experimental groups demonstrated improved performance on upper extremity performance tests most specific to the training performed. However, there were no significant changes on tests of ventilatory muscle performance or simulated activities of daily living.

Celli et al. evaluated thoracic and abdominal respiratory synchrony and transdiaphragmatic pressure during unsupported arm and leg cycle exercise in 12 patients with severe COPD (mean $FEV_1 = 0.68$ liters).[38] They found that arm exercise endurance was significantly less than leg exercise, even though heart rate and oxygen uptake were lower. Also, in the five patients with the most severe obstructive disease, arm exercise was limited by dyspnea and accompanied by dyssynchronous thoracoabdominal breathing. In contrast, in the other seven patients, arm exercise was limited by muscle fatigue and respiratory dyssynchrony did not develop. Respiratory dyssynchrony did not develop in any patient during leg exercise. Maximal transdiaphragmatic pressure decreased similarly in both groups after both arm and leg exercise. The authors suggest that the added burden on the accessory respiratory muscles during upper extremity exercise leads to an increased ventilatory muscle burden, early fatigue, and dyssynchronous breathing, which contributes to the dyspnea observed during such activity. However, this does not appear to be due solely to diaphragmatic fatigue.

In a subsequent study, Criner and Celli compared unsupported and supported arm exercise in 11 patients with severe COPD (mean $FEV_1 = 0.65$ liters).[50] They found that exercise endurance was significantly shorter for unsupported than for supported arm exercise, even though heart rate, ventilation, and oxygen uptake were lower. In examining transdiaphragmatic pressures, the authors then noted that the unsupported arm exercise was associated with a different breathing pattern with a shift of more of the ventilatory load from the inspiratory rib cage muscles to the diaphragm and muscles of expiration.

Ventilatory Muscle. The potential role of ventilatory muscle fatigue as a cause of respiratory failure and ventilatory limitation in patients with COPD has stimulated attempts to train the ventilatory muscles.[37,132] Both isocapnic hyperventilation[21,103] and inspiratory resistive loading[133] have been shown to improve function of these muscles both in healthy subjects and in patients with lung disease. Because respiratory muscle performance does not limit exercise tolerance in healthy subjects, specific respiratory muscle training is unlikely to be of clinical benefit. However, in patients with lung disease who may be limited by respiratory muscles, there may be a role for such training.

Much of the work in this area has focused on patients with COPD. Improvement in exercise performance in patients with COPD from ventilatory muscle training alone has not been demonstrated consistently and the potential role of such training incorporated routinely into pulmonary rehabilitation programs clearly is not established.[40,72,78,132] For instance, Pardy et al. reported that improvement in exercise performance from ventilatory muscle training was present only in a subset of patients with COPD who demonstrated evidence of inspiratory muscle fatigue during exercise.[133] However, at present, there is no simple method to select patients most likely to benefit from this type of exercise training.

Some of the inconsistency in many of the early studies evaluating ventilatory muscle training in patients with COPD may be due to the fact that most of these studies did not control for the inspiratory load during training. Several more recent studies have highlighted the importance of this variable. Larson et al. reported results on 22 patients with COPD who were randomly allocated to train at either 15% or 30% of their maximal inspiratory pressure (MIP) with a threshold pressure breathing device.[101] Only patients who trained at the higher level improved their MIP and endurance time for resistive breathing as well as the distance walked in 12 minutes. However, there were no changes in patients' report of functional impairment, mood, health status, or respiratory symptoms. Harver et al. evaluated targeted inspiratory muscle training to placebo control in 19 patients with COPD and found that the experimental group demonstrated improved maximal inspiratory muscle strength (but not significantly greater than controls) and decreased dyspnea after training.[75]

References

1. Agle DP, Baum GL. Psychological aspects of chronic obstructive pulmonary disease. *Med Clin North Am.* 1977;61:749-758.
2. Agle DP, Baum GL, Chester EH, Wendt M. Multidiscipline treatment of chronic pulmonary insufficiency: 1. Psychologic aspects of rehabilitation. *Psychosom Med.* 1973;35:41-49.
3. Alpert JS, Bass H, Szucs MM, et al. Effects of physical training on hemodynamics and pulmonary function at rest and during exercise in patients with chronic obstructive pulmonary disease. *Chest.* 1975;66:647-651.
4. Ambrosino N, Paggiaro PL, Macchi M, et al. A study of short-term effect of rehabilitative therapy in chronic obstructive pulmonary disease. *Respiration.* 1981;41:40-44.
5. American Thoracic Society. Pulmonary rehabilitation. *Am Rev Respir Dis.* 1981;124:663-666.
6. American Thoracic Society. Standards for the diagnosis and care of patients with chronic obstructive pulmonary disease (COPD) and asthma. *Am Rev Respir Dis.* 1987;136:225-244.
7. Anthonisen NR. Long-term oxygen therapy. *Ann Intern Med.* 1983;99:519-527.
8. Anthonisen NR, Wright EC, Hodgkin JE. Prognosis in chronic obstructive pulmonary disease. *Am Rev Respir Dis.* 1986;133:14-20.
9. Anthonisen P, Riis P, Sogaard-Andersen T. The value of lung physiotherapy in the treatment of acute exacerbations in chronic bronchitis. *Acta Med Scand.* 1964;175:715-719.
10. Ashikaga T, Vacek PM, Lewis SO. Evaluation of a community-based education program for individuals with chronic obstructive pulmonary disease. *J Rehabil Res Dev.* 1980;46:23-27.
11. Atkins CJ, Kaplan RM, Timms RM, Reinsch S, Lofback K. Behavioral exercise programs in the management of chronic obstructive pulmonary disease. *J Consult Clin Psychol.* 1984;52:591-603.
12. Barach AL. Breathing exercises in pulmonary emphysema and allied chronic respiratory disease. *Arch Phys Med Rehabil.* 1955;36:379-390.
13. Barach AL. Physiologic advantages of grunting, groaning, and pursed-lip breathing: adaptive symptoms related to the development of continuous positive pressure breathing. *Bull NY Acad Med.* 1973;49:666-673.
14. Barach AL, Bickerman HA, Beck G. Advances in the treatment of non-tuberculous pulmonary disease. *Bull NY Acad Med.* 1952;28:353-384.
15. Bass H, Whitcomb JF, Forman R. Exercise training: therapy for patients with chronic obstructive pulmonary disease. *Chest.* 1970;57:116-121.

16. Bateman JRM, Newman SP, Daunt KM, Pavia D, Clarke SW. Regional lung clearance of excessive bronchial secretions during chest physiotherapy in patients with stable chronic airways disease. *Lancet.* 1979;1:294-297.

17. Bebout DE, Hodgkin JE, Zorn EG, Yee AR, Sammer EA. Clinical and physiological outcomes of a university-hospital pulmonary rehabilitation program. *Respir Care.* 1983;28:1468-1473.

18. Becklake MR, McGregor M, Goldman HI, Braudo JL. A study of the effects of physiotherapy in chronic hypertrophic emphysema using lung function tests. *Dis Chest.* 1954;26:180-191.

19. Belman MJ. Exercise in chronic obstructive pulmonary disease. *Clin Chest Med.* 1986;7:585-597.

20. Belman MJ, Kendregan BA. Exercise training fails to increase skeletal muscle enzymes in patients with chronic obstructive pulmonary disease. *Am Rev Respir Dis.* 1981;123:256-261.

21. Belman MJ, Mittman C, Weir R. Ventilatory muscle training improves exercise capacity in chronic obstructive pulmonary disease patients. *Am Rev Respir Dis.* 1980;121:273-280.

22. Belman MJ, Wasserman K. Exercise training and testing in patients with chronic obstructive pulmonary disease. *Basics of RD.* 1981;10:1-6.

23. Block AJ. Low flow oxygen therapy: treatment of the ambulant outpatient. *Am Rev Respir Dis.* 1974;110:71-83.

24. Block AJ, Castle JR, Keitt AS. Chronic oxygen therapy: treatment of chronic obstructive pulmonary disease at sea level. *Chest.* 1974;65:279-288.

25. Booker HA. Exercise training and breathing control in patients with chronic airflow limitation. *Physiotherapy.* 1984;70:258-260.

26. Borg GAV. Psychophysical bases of perceived exertion. *Med Sci Sports Exerc.* 1982;14:377-381.

27. Bradley BL, Garner AE, Billiu D, Mestas JM, Forman J. Oxgyen-assisted exercise in chronic obstructive lung disease: the effect on exercise capacity and arterial blood gas tensions. *Am Rev Respir Dis.* 1978;118:239-243.

28. Brown HV, Wasserman K. Exercise performance in chronic obstructive pulmonary diseases. *Med Clin North Am.* 1981;65:525-547.

29. Brundin A. Physical training in severe chronic obstructive lung disease: I. clinical course, physical working capacity and ventilation. *Scand J Respir Dis.* 1974;55:25-36.

30. Buist AS. Acute respiratory infections as a risk factor for chronic airways disease. *Chest.* 1989;96(Suppl):313s-314s.

31. Buist AS. Asthma as a risk factor for chronic airways disease. *Chest.* 1989;96(Suppl):314s-315s.

32. Busch AJ, McClements JD. Effects of a supervised home exercise program on patients with severe chronic obstructive pulmonary disease. *Phys Ther.* 1988;68:469-474.

33. Campbell EJM, Friend J. Action of breathing exercises in pulmonary emphysema. *Lancet.* 1955;268:325-329.

34. Carter R, Nicotra B, Clark L, et al. Exercise conditioning in the rehabilitation of patients with chronic obstructive pulmonary disease. *Arch Phys Med Rehabil.* 1988;69:118-222.

35. Casaburi R, Wasserman K. Exercise training in pulmonary rehabilitation. *N Engl J Med.* 1986;314:1509-1511.

36. Casaburi R, Wasserman K, Patessio A, et al. A new perspective in pulmonary rehabilitation: anaerobic threshold as a discriminant in training. *Eur Respir J.* 1989;2(Suppl 7):618s-623s.

37. Celli BR. Respiratory muscle function. *Clin Chest Med.* 1986;7:567-584.

38. Celli BR, Rassulo J, Make BJ. Dyssynchronous breathing during arm but not leg exercise in patients with chronic airflow obstruction. *N Engl J Med.* 1986;314:1485-1490.

39. Centers for Disease Control. Chronic disease reports: mortality trends—United States, 1979-1986. *MMWR.* 1989;38:189-191.

40. Cherniack RM. Physical therapy techniques. In Hodgkin JE and Petty TL (Eds). *Chronic Obstructive Pulmonary Disease: Current Concepts.* Philadelphia, PA: WB Saunders Co, 1987;113-119.

41. Chester EH, Belman MJ, Bahler RC, et al. Multidisciplinary treatment of chronic pulmonary insufficiency: 3. the effect of physical training on cardiopulmonary performance in patients with chronic obstructive pulmonary disease. *Chest.* 1977;72:695-702.

42. Chretien J. Pollution (atmospheric, domestic, and occupational) as a risk factor for chronic airways disease. *Chest.* 1989;96(Suppl):316s-317s.

43. Christie D. Physical training in chronic obstructive lung disease. *Br Med J.* 1968;2:150-151.

44. Christopher KL, Spofford BT, Petrun MD, et al. A program for transtracheal oxygen delivery: assessment of safety and efficacy. *Ann Intern Med.* 1987;107:802-808.

45. Clausen JL, Zarins LP (Eds). *Pulmonary Function Testing Guidelines and Controversies: Equipment, Methods, and Normal Values.* New York, NY: Academic Press, 1982.

46. Cockcroft A, Berry G, Brown EB, Exall C. Psychological changes during a controlled trial of rehabilitation in chronic respiratory disability. *Thorax.* 1982;37:413-416.

47. Cockcroft AE, Saunders MT, Berry G. Randomised controlled trial of rehabilitation in chronic respiratory disability. *Thorax.* 1981;36:200-203.

48. Connors GA, Hodgkin JE, Asmus RM. A careful assessment is crucial to successful pulmonary rehabilitation. *J Cardiopulmonary Rehabil.* 1988;11:435-438.

49. Cotes JE, Bishop JM, Capel LH, et al. Disabling chest disease: prevention and care: a report of the Royal College of Physicians by the College Committee on Thoracic Medicine. *JR Coll Physicians Lond.* 1981;15:69-87.

50. Criner GJ, Celli BR. Effect of unsupported arm exercise on ventilatory muscle recruitment in patients with severe chronic airflow obstruction. *Am Rev Respir Dis.* 1988;138:856-861.

51. Crofton J, Bjartveit K. Smoking as a risk factor for chronic airways disease. *Chest.* 1989;96(Suppl):307s-312s.

52. Curgian LM, Gronkiewicz CA. Enhancing sexual performance in COPD. *Nurse Practitioner.* 1988;13:34-38.

53. Dales RE, Spitzer WO, Schechter MT, Suissa S. The influence of psychological status on respiratory symptom reporting. *Am Rev Respir Dis.* 1989;139:1459-1463.

54. Daughton DM, Fix AJ, Kas I, Patil KD, Bell CW. Physiological-intellectual components of rehabilitation success in patients with chronic obstructive pulmonary disease (COPD). *J Chron Dis.* 1979;32:405-409.

55. Davidson AC, Leach R, George RJD, Geddes DM. Supplemental oxygen and exercise ability in chronic obstructive airways disease. *Thorax.* 1988;43:965-971.

56. Davies CTM, Sargeant AJ. Effects of training on the physiological responses to one- and two-leg work. *J Appl Physiol.* 1975;38:377-381.

57. DeCencio DV, Leshner B. Personality characteristics of patients with chronic obstructive pulmonary emphysema. *Arch Phys Med Rehabil.* 1968;49:471-475.

58. Dudley DL, Glaser EM, Jorgenson BN, Logan DL. Psychosocial concomitants to rehabilitation in chronic obstructive pulmonary disease: Part 1. Psychosocial and psychological considerations; Part 2. Psychosocial treatment; Part 3. Dealing with psychiatric disease (as distinguishing from psychosocial or psychophysiologic problems). *Chest.* 1980;77:413-420;544-551;677-684.

59. Faling LJ. Pulmonary rehabilitation—physical modalities. *Clin Chest Med.* 1986;7:599-618.

60. Fishman DB, Petty TL. Physical, symptomatic, and psychological improvement in patients receiving comprehensive care for chronic airway obstruction. *J Chronic Dis.* 1971;24:775-785.

61. Fix AJ, Daughton D, Kass I, et al. Personality traits affecting vocational rehabilitation success in patients with chronic obstructive pulmonary disease. *Psych Reports.* 1978;43:939-944.

62. Fletcher C, Peto R, Tinker C, Speizer FE. *The Natural History of Chronic Bronchitis and Emphysema.* Oxford, England: Oxford University Press, 1976.

63. Fletcher EC, Martin RJ. Sexual dysfunction and erectile impotence in chronic obstructive pulmonary disease. *Chest.* 1982;81:413-421.

64. Foster S, Lopez D, Thomas HM. Pulmonary rehabilitation in COPD patients with elevated PCO_2. *Am Rev Respir Dis.* 1988;138:1519-1523.

65. Foster S, Thomas HM. Pulmonary rehabilitation in lung disease other than Chronic Obstructive Pulmonary Disease. *Am Rev Respir Dis.* 1990;141:601-604.

66. Fulme JD, Snider GL. AACP-NHBLI national conference on oxygen therapy. *Chest.* 1984;86:234-247.

67. Gergley TJ, McArdle WD, DeJesus P, et al. Specificity of arm training on aerobic power during swimming and running. *Med Sci Sports Exerc.* 1984;16:349-354.

68. Gilmartin ME. Patient and family education. *Clin Chest Med.* 1986; 7:619-627.

69. Glaser EM, Dudley DL. Psychosocial rehabilitation and psychopharmacology. In Hodgkin JE and Petty TL (Eds). *Chronic Obstructive Pul-*

monary Disease: Current Concepts. Philadelphia, PA: W.B. Saunders Co., 1987;128-153.

70. Goldstein RS, McCullough C, Contreras MA. Approaches to rehabilitation of patients with ventilatory insufficiency. *Eur Respir J.* 1989;2(Suppl 7):655s-660s.

71. Graham WGB, Bradley DA. Efficacy of chest physiotherapy and intermittent positive-pressure breathing in the resolution of pneumonia. *New Engl J Med.* 1978;299:624-627.

72. Grassino A. Inspiratory muscle training in COPD patients. *Eur Respir J.* 1989;2(Suppl 7):581s-586s.

73. Guyatt GH, Berman LB, Townsend M. Long-term outcome after respiratory rehabilitation. *Can Med Assoc J.* 1987;137:1089-1095.

74. Haas A, Cardon H. Rehabilitation in chronic obstructive pulmonary disease: a 5 year study of 252 male patients. *Med Clin North Am.* 1969;53:593-606.

75. Harver A, Mahler DA, Daubenspeck JA. Targeted inspiratory muscle training improves respiratory muscle function and reduces dyspnea in patients with chronic obstructive pulmonary disease. *Ann Intern Med.* 1989;111:117-124.

76. Higgins ITT. Epidemiology of bronchitis and emphysema. In Fishman AP. (Ed). *Pulmonary Diseases and Disorders*, 2nd Edition. New York, NY: McGraw-Hill Book Co., 1988;1237-1246.

77. Higgins MW. Chronic airways disease in the United States: trends and determinants. *Chest.* 1989;96(Suppl):328s-334s.

78. Hodgkin JE. Exercise testing and training. In Hodgkin JE and Petty TL (Eds). *Chronic Obstructive Pulmonary Disease: Current Concepts.* Philadelphia, PA: W.B. Saunders Co., 1987;120-127.

79. Hodgkin JE. Pulmonary rehabilitation. In Hodgkin JE and Petty TL (Eds). *Chronic Obstructive Pulmonary Disease: Current Concepts.* Philadelphia, PA: W.B. Saunders Co., 1987;154-171.

80. Hodgkin JE. Pulmonary rehabilitation: structure, components, and benefits. *J Cardiopulmonary Rehabil.* 1988;11:423-434.

81. Hodgkin JE, Asmus RM, Connors GA. Pulmonary rehabilitation: designing a program that works. *J Respir Dis.* 1987;8:55-68.

82. Hodgkin JE, Balchum OJ, Kass I, et al. Chronic obstructive airway diseases: current concepts in diagnosis and comprehensive care. *JAMA.* 1975;232:1243-1260.

83. Hodgkin JE, Litzau KL. Exercise training target heart rates in chronic obstructive pulmonary disease. *Chest.* 1988;94:30s.

84. Hodgkin JE, Zorn EG, Connors GL (Eds). *Pulmonary Rehabilitation—Guidelines to Success.* Boston, Mass: Butterworth Publishers, 1984.

85. Holland WW. Chronic airways disease in the United Kingdom. *Chest.* 1989;96(Suppl):318s-321s.

86. Holle RHO, Williams DV, Vandree JC, Starks GL, Schoene RB. Increased muscle efficiency and sustained benefits in an outpatient community hospital-based pulmonary rehabilitation program. *Chest.* 1988;94:1161-1168.

87. Hopp JW, Lee JW, Hills R. Development and validation of a pulmonary rehabilitation knowledge test. *J Cardiopulmonary Rehabil.* 1989;7:273-280.

88. Howland J, Nelson EC, Barlow PB, et al. Chronic obstructive airway disease: impact of health education. *Chest.* 1986;90:233-238.

89. Hudson LD, Tyler ML, Petty TL. Hospitalization needs during an outpatient rehabilitation program for severe chronic airway obstruction. *Chest.* 1976;70:606-610.

90. Hughes RL, Davison R. Limitations of exercise reconditioning in COLD. *Chest.* 1983;83:241-249.

91. The Intermittent Positive Pressure Breathing Trial Group. Intermittent positive pressure breathing therapy of chronic obstructive pulmonary disease. *Ann Intern Med.* 1983;99:612-620.

92. Jensen PS. Risk, protective factors, and supportive interventions in chronic airway obstruction. *Arch Gen Psychiatry.* 1983;40:1203-1207.

93. Johnson HR, Tanzi F, Balchum OJ, et al. Inpatient comprehensive pulmonary rehabilitation in severe COPD. *Respir Therapy.* 1980;May/June:15-19.

94. Jones PW, Baveystock CM, Littlejohns P. Relationships between general health measured with the sickness impact profile and respiratory symptoms, physiological measures, and mood in patients with chronic airflow limitation. *Am Rev Respir Dis.* 1989;140:1538-1543.

95. Kaplan RM, Atkins CJ, Timms R. Validity of a quality of well-being scale as an outcome measure in chronic obstructive pulmonary disease. *J Chron Dis.* 1984;37:85-95.

96. Kaplan RM, Ries A, Atkins CJ. Behavioral management of chronic obstructive pulmonary disease. *Ann Behav Med.* 1985;7:5-10.

97. Kass I, Dyksterhuis JE, Rubin H, Patil KD. Correlation of psychophysiological variables with vocational rehabilitation outcome in patients with chronic obstructive pulmonary disease. *Chest.* 1975;67:433-440.

98. Kimbel P, Kaplan AS, Alkalay I, Lester D. An inhospital program for rehabilitation of patients with chronic obstructive pulmonary disease. *Chest.* 1971;60(Suppl):6s-10s.

99. Kirilloff LH, Carpenter V, Kerby GR, Kigin C, Weimer MP. Skills of the health team involved in out-of-hospital care for patients with COPD. *Am Rev Respir Dis.* 1986;133:948-949.

100. Kirilloff LH, Owens GR, Rogers RM, Mazzocco MC. Does chest physical therapy work? *Chest.* 1985;88:436-444.

101. Larson JL, Kim MJ, Sharp JT, Larson DA. Inspiratory muscle training with a pressure threshold breathing device in patients with chronic obstructive pulmonary disease. *Am Rev Respir Dis.* 1988;138:689-696.

102. Lefcoe NM, Paterson NAM. Adjunct therapy in chronic obstructive pulmonary disease. *Am J Med.* 1973;54:343-350.

103. Leith DE, Bradley M. Ventilatory muscle strength and endurance training. *J Appl Physiol.* 1976;41:508-516.

104. Lenfant C. Lung research: government and community. *Am Rev Respir Dis.* 1982;126:753-757.

105. Lertzman MM, Cherniack RM. Rehabilitation of patients with chronic obstructive pulmonary disease. *Am Rev Respir Dis.* 1976;114:1145-1165.

106. Light RW, Merrill EJ, Despars JA, Gordon GH, Mutalipassi LR. Prevalence of depression and anxiety in patients with COPD: relationship to functional capacity. *Chest.* 1985;87:35-38.

107. Longo AM, Moser KM, Luchsinger PC. The role of oxygen therapy in rehabilitation of patients with chronic obstructive pulmonary disease. *Am Rev Respir Dis.* 1971;103:690-697.

108. Lustig FM, Haas A, Castillo R. Clinical and rehabilitation regime in patients with chronic

obstructive pulmonary disease. *Arch Phys Med Rehabil.* 1972;53:315-322.

109. Magel JR, McArdle WD, Toner M, Delio DJ. Metabolic and cardiovascular adjustment to arm training. *J Appl Physiol.* 1978;45:75-79.

110. Make BJ (Ed). Pulmonary rehabilitation. *Clin Chest Med.* 1986;7:519-702.

111. Mall RW, Medeiros M. Objective evaluation of results of a pulmonary rehabilitation program in a community hospital. *Chest.* 1988;94:1156-1160.

112. McGavin CR, Gupta SP, Lloyd EL, McHardy JR. Physical rehabilitation of chronic bronchitis: results of a controlled trial of exercises in the home. *Thorax.* 1977;32:307-311.

113. McSweeny AJ, Grant I, Heaton RK, Adams KM, Timms RM. Life quality of patients with chronic obstructive pulmonary disease. *Arch Intern Med.* 1982;142:473-478.

114. Medical Research Council Working Party. Long-term domicillary oxygen therapy in chronic hypoxic cor pulmonale complicating chronic bronchitis and emphysema. *Lancet.* 1981;1:681-686.

115. Mertens DJ, Shephard RJ, Kavanagh T. Long-term exercise therapy for chronic obstructive lung disease. *Respiration.* 1978;35:96-107.

116. Meuller RE, Kebe DL, Plummer J, Walker SH. The prevalence of chronic bronchitis, chronic airway obstruction, and respiratory symptoms in a Colorado city. *Am Rev Respir Dis.* 1971;103:209-228.

117. Miller WF. A physiologic evaluation of the effects of diaphragmatic breathing training in patients with chronic pulmonary emphysema. *Am J Med.* 1954;17:471-477.

118. Miller WF. Physical therapeutic measures in the treatment of chronic bronchopulmonary disorders: methods for breathing training. *Am J Med.* 1958;24:929-940.

119. Mohsenifar Z, Horak D, Brown HV, Koerner SK. Sensitive indices of improvement in a pulmonary rehabilitation program. *Chest.* 1983;83:189-192.

120. Moser KM, Archibald C, Hansen P, Ellis B, Whelan D. *Shortness of Breath—A Guide to Better Living and Breathing.* 3rd ed. St. Louis, MO: CV Mosby, 1983.

121. Moser KM, Bokinsky GE, Savage RT, Archibald CJ, Hansen PR. Results of a comprehensive rehabilitation program: physiologic and functional effects on patients with chronic obstructive pulmonary disease. *Arch Intern Med.* 1980;140:1596-1601.

122. Motley HL. The effects of slow deep breathing on the blood gas exchange in emphysema. *Am Rev Respir Dis.* 1963;88:484-492.

123. Mueller RE, Petty TL, Filley GF. Ventilation and arterial blood gas changes induced by pursed lips breathing. *J Appl Physiol.* 1970;28:784-789.

124. Mungall IPF, Hainsworth R. Assessment of respiratory function in patients with chronic obstructive airways disease. *Thorax.* 1979;34:254-258.

125. Murray JF (Ed). Chronic airways disease—distribution and determinants, prevention and control. *Chest.* 1989;96(Suppl):301s-378s.

126. Neish CM, Hopp JW. The role of education in pulmonary rehabilitation. *J Cardiopulmonary Rehabil.* 1988;11:439-441.

127. Nicholas JJ, Gilbert R, Gabe R, Auchincloss JH. Evaluation of an exercise therapy program for patients with chronic obstructive pulmonary disease. *Am Rev Respir Dis.* 1970;102:1-9.

128. Nicol J, Hodgkin JE, Connors G, et al. Strategies for developing a cost-effective pulmonary rehabilitation program. *Respir Care.* 1983;28:1451-1455.

129. Nocturnal Oxygen Therapy Trial Group. Continuous or nocturnal oxygen therapy in hypoxemic chronic obstructive lung disease: a clinical trial. *Ann Intern Med.* 1980;93:391-398.

130. Paez PN, Phillipson EA, Masangkay M, Sproule BJ. The physiologic basis of training patients with emphysema. *Am Rev Respir Dis.* 1967;95:944-953.

131. Paine R, Make BJ. Pulmonary rehabilitation for the elderly. *Clin Geriatr Med.* 1986;2:313-335.

132. Pardy RL, Reid WD, Belman MJ. Respiratory muscle training. *Clin Chest Med.* 1988;9:287-296.

133. Pardy RL, Rivington RN, Despas PJ, Macklem PT. The effects of inspiratory muscle training on exercise performance in chronic airflow limitation. *Am Rev Respir Dis.* 1981;123:426-433.

134. Paul G, Eldridge F, Mitchell J, Fiene T. Some effects of slowing respiration rate in chronic emphysema and bronchitis. *J Appl Physiol.* 1966;21:877-882.

135. Petty TL. The national mucolytic study: results of a randomized, double-blind, placebo-controlled study of iodinated glycerol in chronic obstructive bronchitis. *Chest.* 1990; 97:75-83.

136. Petty TL, Finigan MM. Clinical evaluation of prolonged ambulatory oxygen therapy in chronic airway obstruction. *Am J Med.* 1968;45:242-252.

137. Petty TL, MacIlroy ER, Swigert MA, Brink GA. Chronic airway obstruction, respiratory insufficiency, and gainful employment. *Arch Environ Health.* 1970;21:71-78.

138. Petty TL, Nett LM, Finigan MM, Brink GA, Corsello PR. A comprehensive care program for chronic airway obstruction: methods and preliminary evaluation of symptomatic and functional improvement. *Ann Intern Med.* 1969;70:1109-1120.

139. Pierce AK, Taylor HF, Archer RK, Miller WF. Responses to exercise training in patients with emphysema. *Arch Intern Med.* 1964;113:28-36.

140. Prigatano GP, Wright EC, Levin D. Quality of life and its predictors in patients with mild hypoxemia and chronic obstructive pulmonary disease. *Arch Intern Med.* 1984;144:1613-1619.

141. Pryor JA, Webber BA, Hodson ME, Batten JC. Evaluation of the forced expiration technique as an adjunct to postural drainage in treatment of cystic fibrosis. *Br Med J.* 1979;2:417-418.

142. Reisman JJ, Rivington-Law B, Corey M, et al. Role of conventional physiotherapy in cystic fibrosis. *J Pediatr.* 1988;113:632-636.

143. Renfroe KL. Effect of progressive relaxation on dyspnea and state anxiety in patients with chronic obstructive pulmonary disease. *Heart Lung.* 1988;17:408-413.

144. Renzetti AD, Jr, McClement JH, Litt BD. The Veterans Administration cooperative study of pulmonary function: III. mortality in relation to respiratory function in chronic obstructive pulmonary disease. *Am J Med.* 1966;41:115-129.

145. Reybrouck T, Heigenhauser GF, Faulkner JA. Limitations to maximum oxygen uptake in arm, leg, and combined arm-leg ergometry. *J Appl Physiol.* 1975;38:774-779.

146. Ries AL. Pulmonary rehabilitation. In Fishman AP (Ed). *Pulmonary Diseases and Disorders.* 2nd ed. New York, NY: McGraw-Hill Book Co., 1988;1325-1331.

147. Ries AL. The role of exercise testing in pulmonary diagnosis. *Clinics Chest Med.* 1987;8:81-89.

148. Ries AL, Archibald CJ. Endurance exercise training at maximal targets in patients with chronic obstructive pulmonary disease. *J Cardiopulmonary Rehabil.* 1987;7:594-601.

149. Ries AL, Ellis B, Hawkins RW. Upper extremity exercise training in chronic obstructive pulmonary disease. *Chest.* 1988;93:688-692.

150. Ries AL, Farrow JT, Clausen JL. Accuracy of two ear oximeters at rest and during exercise in pulmonary patients. *Am Rev Respir Dis.* 1985;132:685-689.

151. Ries AL, Farrow JT, Clausen JL. Pulmonary function tests cannot predict exercise-induced hypoxemia in chronic obstructive pulmonary disease. *Chest.* 1988;93:454-459.

152. Ries AL, Moser KM. Predicting treadmill/walking speed from cycle ergometry exercise in chronic obstructive pulmonary disease. *Am Rev Respir Dis.* 1982;126:924-927.

153. Rochester DF, Goldberg SK. Techniques of respiratory physical therapy. *Am Rev Respir Dis.* 1980;122(Suppl):133-146.

154. Sackner MA, Silva G, Banks JM, Watson DD, Smoak WM. Distribution of ventilation during diaphragmatic breathing in obstructive lung disease. *Am Rev Respir Dis.* 1974;109:331-337.

155. Sahn SA, Nett LM, Petty TL. Ten-year follow-up of a comprehensive rehabilitation program for severe COPD. *Chest.* 1980;77:311-314.

156. Saltin B, Nazar K, Costill DL, et al. The nature of the training response; peripheral and central adaptations to one-legged exercise. *Acta Physiol Scand.* 1976;96:289-305.

157. Sandhu HS. Psychosocial issues in chronic obstructive pulmonary disease. *Clin Chest Med.* 1986;7:629-642.

158. Sergysels R, Willeput R, Lenders D, et al. Low frequency breathing at rest and during exercise in severe chronic obstructive bronchitis. *Thorax.* 1979;34:536-539.

159. Sexton DL. Relaxation techniques and biofeedback. In Hogkin JE and Petty TL (Eds). *Chronic Obstructive Pulmonary Disease: Current Concepts.* Philadelphia, PA: W.B. Saunders Co., 1987;99-112.

160. Shephard RJ. On the design and effectiveness of training regimens in chronic obstructive lung disease. *Bull Eur Physiopathol Respir.* 1977;13:457-469.

161. Sinclair DJM, Ingram CG. Controlled trial of supervised exercise training in chronic bronchitis. *Br Med J.* 1980;280:519-521.

162. Sinclair JD. The effect of breathing exercises in pulmonary emphysema. *Thorax.* 1955;10:246-249.

163. Sneider R, O'Malley JA, Kahn M. Trends in pulmonary rehabilitation at Eisenhower Medical Center: an 11-years' experience (1976-1987). *J Cardiopulmonary Rehabil.* 1988;11:453-461.

164. Stamford BA, Cuddihee RW, Moffatt RJ, Rowland P. Task specific changes in maximal oxygen uptake resulting from arm versus leg training. *Ergonomics.* 1978;21:1-9.

165. Strijbos JH, Koeter GH, Meinesz AF. Home care rehabilitation and perception of dyspnea in chronic obstructive pulmonary disease (COPD) patients. *Chest.* 1990;97:109s-110s.

166. Sutton PP. Chest physiotherapy: time for reappraisal. *Br J Dis Chest.* 1988;82:127-137.

167. Sutton PP, Gemmell HG, Innes N, et al. Use of nebulised saline and nebulised terbutaline as an adjunct to chest physiotherapy. *Thorax.* 1988;43:57-60.

168. Sutton PP, Parker RA, Webber BA, et al. Assessment of the forced expiration technique, postural drainage and directed coughing in chest physiotherapy. *Eur J Respir Dis.* 1983;64:62-68.

169. Sutton PP, Pavia D, Bateman JRM, Clarke SW. Chest physiotherapy: a review. *Eur J Respir Dis.* 1982;63:188-201.

170. Tandon MK. Adjunct treatment with yoga in chronic severe airways obstruction. *Thorax.* 1978;33:514-517.

171. Tangri S, Woolf CR. The breathing pattern in chronic obstructive lung disease during the performance of some common daily activities. *Chest.* 1973;63:126-127.

172. *The Health Consequences of Smoking: Chronic Obstructive Lung Disease: A Report of the Surgeon General.* Rockville, MD: Department of Health and Human Services, PHS Office on Smoking and Health, 1984.

173. *The Health Consequences of Smoking: Cardiovascular Disease: A Report of the Surgeon General.* Rockville, MD: Department of Health and Human Services, PHS Office on Smoking and Health, 1983.

174. Thoman RL, Stoker GL, Ross JC. The efficacy of pursed-lips breathing in patients with

chronic obstructive pulmonary disease. *Am Rev Respir Dis.* 1966;93:100-106.

175. Tiep BL. Oxygen therapy for the mobile patient. *J Cardiopulmonary Rehabil.* 1988;11:442-448.

176. Tiep BL, Burns M, Kao D, Madison R, Herrera J. Pursed lips breathing training using ear oximetry. *Chest.* 1986;90:218-221.

177. Tiep BL, Lewis MI. Oxygen conservation and oxygen-conserving devices in chronic lung disease: a review. *Chest.* 1987;92:263-272.

178. Timms RM. Sexual dysfunction and chronic obstructive pulmonary disease. *Chest.* 1982;81:398-400.

179. Traver GA. Measures of symptoms and life quality to predict emergent use of institutional health care resources in chronic obstructive airways disease. *Heart Lung.* 1988;17:689-697.

180. Traver GA, Cline MG, Burrows B. Predictors of mortality in chronic obstructive pulmonary disease: a 15-year follow-up study. *Am Rev Respir Dis.* 1979;119:895-902.

181. Tydeman DE, Chandler AR, Graveling BM, Culot A, Harrison BDW. An investigation into the effects of exercise tolerance training on patients with chronic airways obstruction. *Physiotherapy.* 1984;70:261-264.

182. Vokac Z, Bell H, Bautz-Holter E, Rodahl K. Oxygen uptake/heart rate relationship in leg and arm exercise, sitting and standing. *J Appl Physiol.* 1975;39:54-59.

183. Vyas MN, Banister EW, Morton JW, Grzybowski S. Response to exercise in patients with chronic airway obstruction: I. effects of exercise training. *Am Rev Respir Dis.* 1971;103:390-400.

184. Vyas MN, Banister EW, Morton JW, Grzybowski S. Response to exercise in patients with chronic airway obstruction: II. effects of breathing 40 percent oxygen. *Am Rev Respir Dis.* 1971;103:401-412.

185. Wasserman K, Sue DY, Casaburi R, Moricca RB. Selection criteria for exercise training in pulmonary rehabilitation. *Eur Respir J.* 1989;2(Suppl 7):604s-610s.

186. White B, Andrews JL, Jr, Mogan JJ, Downes-Vogel P. Pulmonary rehabilitation in an ambulatory group practice setting. *Med Clin North Am.* 1979;63:379-390.

187. Williams IP, Smith CM, McGavin CR. Diaphragmatic breathing training and walking performance in chronic airways obstruction. *Br J Dis Chest.* 1982;76:164-166.

188. Williams SJ. Chronic respiratory illness and disability: a critical review of the psychosocial literature. *Soc Sci Med.* 1989;28:791-803.

189. Wilson AF. *Pulmonary Function Testing Indications and Interpretations.* Orlando, Fla.: Grune & Stratton, 1985.

190. Woolcock AJ. Epidemiology of chronic airways disease. *Chest.* 1989;96(Suppl):302s-306s.

191. Woolf CR, Suero JT. Alterations in lung mechanics and gas exchange following training in chronic obstructive lung disease. *Dis Chest.* 1969;55:37-44.

192. Zack MB, Palange AV. Oxygen supplemented exercise of ventilatory and nonventilatory muscles in pulmonary rehabilitation. *Chest.* 1985; 88:669-675.

American Thoracic Society Official Statement on Pulmonary Rehabilitation

This official ATS statement was adopted by the ATS Executive Committee, March 1981.

Introduction

The purpose of this statement is to define pulmonary rehabilitation and to describe the essential elements of a pulmonary rehabilitation program. In order to provide comprehensive pulmonary rehabilitation services, a program should be able to carry out the described components of pulmonary rehabilitation and to provide the essential services required as defined in this statement.

Definition of Pulmonary Rehabilitation

Rehabilitation was defined by the Council of Rehabilitation in 1942 as the restoration of the individual to the fullest medical, mental, emotional, social, and vocational potential of which he/she is capable. Instead of addressing solely the physical and mental aspects, rehabilitation should be tailored to maximize one's improvement and minimize the impact of an illness, or a state of progressive deterioration from optimal health, not only on the person, but also his/her family and community.

The American College of Chest Physicians' Committee on Pulmonary Rehabilitation adopted, at its annual meeting in 1974, the following definition:

Pulmonary rehabilitation may be defined as an art of medical practice wherein an individually tailored, multidisciplinary program is formulated which through accurate diagnosis, therapy, emotional support, and education, stabilizes or reverses both the physio- and psychopathology of pulmonary diseases and attempts to return the patient to the highest possible functional capacity allowed by his pulmonary handicap and overall life situation.

The two principal objectives of pulmonary rehabilitation are to: (1) control and alleviate as much as possible the symptoms and pathophysiologic complications of respiratory impairment, and (2) teach the patient how to achieve optimal capability for carrying out his/her activities of daily living. Depending on the needs of the specific patient, comprehensive care may include the delivery of a structured, defined "rehabilitation program" as an element of the patient's care. However, in the broadest sense, pulmonary rehabilitation means providing good, comprehensive respiratory care for patients with pulmonary disease. A facility caring for such individuals should be capable of either providing or having access to a regional medical center that is able to offer such a comprehensive care program. The components of pulmonary rehabilitation described in this statement are most useful for patients with chronic

Note. Reprinted from "Official ATS Statement—Pulmonary Rehabilitation" by the American Lung Association, 1981, *American Review of Respiratory Disease,* **124**:663-666. Copyright 1981 by the American Lung Association.

obstructive pulmonary disease (COPD), e.g., emphysema, chronic bronchitis, and asthma. However, certain aspects may be selected for patients with other pulmonary disorders.

Sequence of Pulmonary Rehabilitation

A certain sequence should be followed when outlining an appropriate treatment plan. This process involves careful evaluation of the patient, developing a treatment program that best meets the patient's needs, proper assessment of the patient's progress, and a plan for patient follow-up. A logical sequence would proceed as follows:

(A) Patient Selection

Any patient with symptomatic COPD should be considered for pulmonary rehabilitation. Those patients with either very mild or very severe disease will not generally be placed on as intensive and comprehensive a rehabilitation program as those with moderate to moderately-severe disease.

Multiple factors affect the ultimate success of rehabilitation for any individual. These include, in addition to severity of the disease, the presence of other disabling diseases such as cancer or arthritis, age, intelligence, level of education, occupation, family support, and personal motivation.

(B) Evaluation

A careful assessment of the patient should be performed initially. This evaluation would include:

(1) Diagnostic Workup

Proper identification of the patient's specific respiratory ailment is important because the treatment regimen prescribed should be geared to the patient's disease process. Essential diagnostic information would include: appropriate pulmonary function studies, a chest radiograph, an electrocardiogram, and, when indicated, arterial blood gas measurements at rest and during exercise, sputum analysis and blood theophylline measurements.

(2) Behavioral Considerations

The best rehabilitation results require personal commitment from the patient, determination and persistence. Additionally, significant psychiatric symptoms of any sort profoundly disrupt compliance. For these reasons, the patient should receive emotional screening assessments and treatment or counseling when required.

Thorough understanding of the disease and its treatment is one of the more important factors in patient motivation, cooperation, and anxiety reduction. This is particularly true in pulmonary rehabilitation during which the patient must master a large amount of knowledge. Yet learning abilities among these patients are often subtly impaired. This can be remedied in two ways: (a) estimating the patient's learning skills and adjusting the program to the patient's ability, and (b) requiring the patient to demonstrate new knowledge and skills before progressing further.

The patient must be viewed in terms of the personal and environmental assets at his/her disposal. These include family and social support, potential employment skills, employment opportunities, and community resources. These all need to be evaluated and mobilized for practical help to the patient and to bolster his/her motivation.

(C) Determine Goals

It is crucial that short- and long-term goals be developed for each individual following the evaluation. The patient and his/her family need to help determine and fully understand these goals, so that they realistically approach the treatment phase.

(D) Components of Pulmonary Rehabilitation

(1) Physical Therapy

Good bronchial hygiene, e.g., effective coughing, clapping, and bronchial drainage is particularly important to those patients who produce excess mucus within the airways. Pursed-lip breathing may help to slow the respiratory rate and lessen small airway collapse during periods of increased dyspnea. Relaxation techniques can be useful in anxious patients.

(2) Exercise Conditioning

A physical conditioning (exercise) program should be considered in any patient with exercise limitations. Selection of appropriate, safe exercise routines is enhanced by measuring workloads, gas exchange behavior, heart rate, and electrocardiogram. However, in selected patients, assessment of the functional work capacity may be possible with such techniques as determining the number of steps the individual can climb or the distance the patient can walk at a certain speed.

(3) Respiratory Therapy

Supplemental oxygen and aerosolization of medications such as bronchodilators and corticosteroids are useful for certain patients. In an attempt to limit the inappropriate and excess use of oxygen and respiratory therapy equipment in the home, the American Thoracic Society has developed statements regarding these treatment modalities.

(4) Education

If patient compliance is to be optimized, both the patient and his/her family need to understand the underlying pulmonary disorder. Those individuals outlining the treatment plan should instruct the patient and family about the purpose for medications, as well as their side effects. Proper nutrition, the use and cleaning of respiratory therapy equipment, techniques of physical therapy modalities, and details of an exercise conditioning program must all be carefully explained.

(5) General

The importance of smoking cessation must be emphasized. Attention should be paid to such environmental factors as temperature, humidity, inhaled irritants, and altitude. Although there is little objective data that adequate hydration liquefies airway secretions, it is agreed that dehydration should be prevented. Immunization with the influenza and pneumococcal vaccines is recommended. An appropriate use of such pharmacologic agents as beta$_2$ agonists, methylxanthines, antimicrobials, and corticosteroids is important, and their indications must be understood by the primary care physician.

(E) Assessment of Patient's Progress

While the treatment plan is being developed, the patient's progress should be monitored. This will help both the patient and the health care team objectively evaluate the plan outlined, so that any needed changes can be initiated.

(F) Long-Term Follow-Up

Ongoing care will generally be the responsibility of the primary care physician. Periodic reassessment can be beneficial to the patient, as a way of objectively evaluating progress and allowing for educational reinforcement.

Services Required for Pulmonary Rehabilitation

A variety of services are provided through a pulmonary rehabilitation program. Many patients with COPD will not need these services; however, they should be available for those patients with special needs or more severe disease.

(A) Essential Services

(1) Initial Medical Evaluation and Care Plan

Perform a complete history and physical examination. Obtain appropriate laboratory tests. Make the correct diagnosis. Outline a proper therapy regimen for ongoing care.

(2) Patient Education, Evaluation, and Program Coordination

Educate patient regarding lung anatomy and physiology, disease process, useful therapeutic modalities, and other relevant matters. Coordinate allied health personnel involved in the patient's care. Make home visits, as necessary.

(3) Respiratory Therapy Techniques

Educate patient concerning proper use and cleaning of respiratory therapy equipment. Administer therapy as prescribed by attending physician. Make home visits as needed to insure compliance.

(4) Physical Therapy Techniques, Including Exercise Conditioning

Educate patient regarding relaxation techniques, proper breathing, clapping, and bronchial drainage. Measure functional work capacity and develop an exercise conditioning program. Record physiologic changes resulting from exercise training.

(5) Daily Performance Evaluation

Evaluate activities of daily living. Teach energy conservation (work simplification) and self-care techniques.

(6) Social Service Evaluation

Obtain social history and determine patient's psychosocial assets and needs. Evaluate potential for compliance as well as actual compliance. Mobilize family or other interested individuals as part of extended support system to be used following discharge from the hospital. Evaluate third-party payor problems and help in resolving such problems. Assist in making arrangements for needed community resources, including financial aid, homemaker services, and extended care facilities.

(7) Nutritional Evaluation

Evaluate the patient's nutritional status. Outline dietary prescription based on the patient's specific nutritional needs.

(B) Additional Services

(1) Psychological Evaluation

Administer psychometric battery that includes tests designed to measure organic brain dysfunction, IQ, personality profile, psychosocial assets, impact of illness on person, his/her family, etc. Help patient and family develop coping mechanisms to control not only chronic anxiety or depression but also acute exacerbations.

(2) Psychiatric Evaluation

Categorize personality pattern. Make psychiatric diagnosis if one exists. Provide specific psychiatric support and/or therapy when needed. If necessary, make specific recommendations regarding optimal psychopharmacologic agents.

(3) Vocational Evaluation

Assess vocational rehabilitation potential for those patients with significant impairment. Includes vocational tests, interviews, on-the-job observation, as well as determining whether the subject has the work capacity to meet the oxygen requirements of his/her job. Work output can generally be sustained for an eight-hour period if one does not exceed 30%-40% of his/her attained maximum oxygen consumption.

A physician knowledgeable about respiratory diseases should perform the initial complete examination and assist in outlining a proper regimen of treatment.

The specific provider for the other services may vary from program to program. A multidisciplinary team that might include a professional nurse, respiratory therapist, physical therapist, occupa-

tional therapist, dietitian, social worker, and pulmonary or cardiopulmonary technologist expert in pulmonary rehabilitation techniques is appropriate for those settings where large numbers of patients are referred and for teaching or research purposes. However, in other settings, it may be possible to provide similar services with fewer individuals if they are highly qualified and specially trained in evaluation and management of the patient with COPD. In selected patients, the evaluation and delivery of a comprehensive care program can be accomplished in an outpatient setting. Thus, the techniques of rehabilitation should be within the reach of all physicians, applying the principles expressed in this document.

Benefits and Limitations of Pulmonary Rehabilitation

(A) Benefits

A comprehensive respiratory care program can result in definite benefits to the patient. There is overwhelming evidence that a comprehensive respiratory care program can result in an improved quality of life and a significantly improved capability for carrying out his/her daily activities.

Participation in a comprehensive pulmonary rehabilitation program has repeatedly been shown to decrease the hospital days required per patient per year. Some patients may be able to return to useful employment, thus making a contribution to the work force. Patients can achieve a significant reduction in anxiety, depression, and somatic concern with an associated improvement in their own ego strength. Numerous studies have shown that the physical conditioning of patients with COPD can be substantially improved with a regular exercise training program.

Cessation of smoking can result in improved pulmonary function, reduction of cough, decreased sputum production, and lessened dyspnea. The course of COPD may be altered if the airway abnormality is detected early.

(B) Limitations

Even though all of the above benefits have been documented, an extension of lifespan and slowing of pulmonary function deterioration have not been shown in the majority of published studies. Through the use of routine office spirometry,

COPD can be detected at a much earlier stage when institution of a comprehensive respiratory care program may more effectively achieve an alteration in the patient's course.

A significant problem relates to the fact that only approximately 20%-35% of the participants in smoking cessation programs quit permanently. More effort needs to be applied to the prevention of respiratory disease, rather than concentrating on treatment after significant disability has occurred.

Another major factor interfering with delivery of good care is the unevenness in our capacity to deliver community-based services. A visiting nurse association (or its equivalent) does not exist in every community, nor do socially-oriented service programs, such as Meals on Wheels, Homemaker's, etc.

Which tests are required to appropriately determine impairment/disability needs to be more clearly determined. Ideally, patients should be adequately evaluated and treated comprehensively *prior to* a final disability determination.

Conclusion

In the 17th century, Jeremy Taylor said, "To preserve a man alive in the midst of so many diseases and hostilities, is as great a miracle as to create him." In the past, rehabilitation has been applied rather loosely to vaguely describe various approaches to long-term management of the chronically ill patient. The time has come for us to not only define what we mean by pulmonary rehabilitation but to describe the essential services required. This comprehensive approach to patient evaluation will result in improved care for respiratory patients so that they may be restored to their most optimal potential.

This statement was prepared by an *ad hoc* committee of the Scientific Assembly on Clinical Problems. The committee members are as follows:

John E. Hodgkin, *Chairman*
Michael J. Farrell
Suzanne R. Gibson
Richard E. Kanner
Irving Kass
Lawrence M. Lampton
Margaret Nield
Thomas L. Petty

References

1. Masferrer R, O'Donohue WJ Jr., Seriff NS, et al. Home use of equipment for patients with respiratory disease [ATS Statement]. *Am Rev Respir Dis.* 1977;115:893-5.

2. Block AJ, Burrows B, Kanner RE, et al. Oxygen administration in the home [ATS Statement]. *Am Rev Respir Dis.* 1977;115:897-9.

3. California Thoracic Society guidelines for pulmonary rehabilitation, a statement by the CTS Respiratory Care Assembly. Newsletter, Respiratory Care Assembly of California Thoracic Society, September 1979, 8(#1).

4. Daughton DM, Fix AJ, Kass I, et al. Physiological-intellectual components of rehabilitation success in patients with chronic obstructive pulmonary disease (COPD). *J Chronic Dis.* 1979;32:405-9.

5. Hodgkin JE, ed. *Chronic Obstructive Pulmonary Disease. Current Concepts in Diagnosis and Comprehensive Care.* Park Ridge, Ill: American College of Chest Physicians, 1979.

6. Hodgkin JE. Pulmonary rehabilitation. In: Simmons D, ed, *Current Pulmonology III.* New York, NY: John Wiley & Sons, 1981.

7. Intermittent positive pressure breathing (IPPB). *Clin Notes Respir Dis.* Winter 1979;3-6.

8. Kimbel P, Kaplan AS, Alkalay I, et al. An in-hospital program for rehabilitation of patients with chronic obstructive pulmonary disease. *Chest.* 1971;60(Suppl):6s-10s.

9. Lertzman MM, Cherniack RM. Rehabilitation of patients with chronic obstructive pulmonary disease. *Am Rev Respir Dis.* 1976;114:1145-65.

10. Moser KM, Bokinsky GE, Savage RT, Archibald CJ, Hansen PR. Physiological and functional effects of a comprehensive rehabilitation program upon patients with chronic obstructive pulmonary disease. *Arch Int Med.* 1980;140:1596-1601.

11. Nield M. The effect of health teaching on the anxiety level of patients with chronic obstructive lung disease. *Nursing Res.* 1971;20:537-41.

12. Petty TL, ed. *Chronic Obstructive Pulmonary Disease.* New York, NY: Marcel Dekker, 1978.

13. Petty TL. *Pulmonary Rehabilitation, Basics of RD.* New York, NY: American Thoracic Society, 1975.

14. Pierce AK, Paez PN, Miller WF. Exercise therapy with the aid of a portable oxygen supply

in patients with emphysema. *Am Rev Respir Dis.* 1965;91:653-9.

15. Skills of the Health Team Involved in Out-of-Hospital Care for Patients with COPD, a statement by the Section on Nursing, Scientific Assembly on Clinical Problems, American Thoracic Society. *ATS News.* 1977;3:18.

Case Studies of Pulmonary Rehabilitation

Case Study 1

Trina M. Limberg, BS, RRT, RCP

Medical History

A 56-year-old white female with chronic obstructive pulmonary disease (COPD) presented to pulmonary rehabilitation for evaluation because of progressive shortness of breath on exertion.

She was in good health until age 42, when she first noted breathlessness with exertion, although she was not diagnosed until age 48. She then began treatment with theophylline, and a B_2 sympathomimetic metered dose inhaler (MDI). She had a 45-pack-per-year smoking history but quit upon diagnosis. Serum alpha-1 antitrypsin levels were within normal limits. There was no history of occupational exposure, childhood illnesses, asthma, or allergies. Family history was unremarkable for pulmonary disease. She was first hospitalized at age 55 for an exacerbation of COPD with a $PaCO_2$ of 49 mmHg and a PaO_2 of 39 on room air. She did not require mechanical ventilation or intubation. She was treated with intravenous antibiotics, corticosteroids, and theophylline as well as respiratory care. After 4 days she was discharged on 2 L/min continuous oxygen therapy; prednisone 40 mg daily and taper as directed; theophylline 300 mg by mouth 3 times a day; and Albuterol MDI two puffs every 3 to 4 hours.

Sometime after attending a community seminar on pulmonary rehabilitation, the patient contacted a pulmonologist, the medical director of the rehabilitation program, for a second opinion. At that time the patient complained of a chronic productive cough since the hospitalization, as well as increasing breathlessness and fatigue. She expressed concern about her rather recent loss of function and described herself as nervous and anxious. Her exercise tolerance was approximately one block. She continued to take the same medications with the addition of an Ipratropium MDI two puffs 4 times a day. Oxygen therapy was being used as needed and at night.

Before the rehabilitation evaluation was completed, the patient's condition deteriorated, resulting in admission to intensive care, where she was intubated and placed on mechanical ventilation for treatment of respiratory failure. After 10 days the patient was weaned, and later she was transferred out of intensive care. She continued to recover gradually. Due to the patient's increased weakness and a reduced ability to ambulate, a home health nurse was arranged for support after discharge.

Evaluation for Pulmonary Rehabilitation

Patient evaluation involved a complete review of her medical history, including past medical history, current medications, and social history.

Past Medical History

Remarkable for rheumatic fever at age 8 treated with bed rest for 1 year. She had a skin cancer removed from the right side of her neck several years ago. She reported an allergy to codeine. There was no history of hypertension, cardiac disease, or bone or joint problems.

Current Medications

Theophylline: 300 mg twice a day
Albuterol: MDI 2 puffs every 4 hours and as needed
Ipratroprium: MDI 2 puffs every 4 hours
Beclomethasone: MDI 4 puffs 4 times a day
Xanax: .25 mg as needed for anxiety
Oxygen therapy: 2 L/min as needed

Social History

She was born in New York state, lived in cities in the East, and eventually settled on the West coast. She was married for 37 years and had three grown children who were alive and well. She worked for a publishing company with an office job for 12 years and stopped after her hospitalization because of her health.

Assessment

During the initial interview and assessment with the rehabilitation staff, the following problems were identified:

- Decreased exercise tolerance
- Poor compliance with continuous oxygen therapy prescription
- Reduced strength in upper and lower extremities
- Dyspnea with all activities of daily living
- Poor knowledge and understanding of disease process, management, and treatment
- Ineffective breathing and coughing techniques
- Improper use of metered dose inhaler
- Inability to self-assess and report symptom changes early
- Anxiety and panic episodes
- Lack of energy-saving and pacing skills

Diagnostic Tests for Pulmonary Rehabilitation

Following the initial assessment, the patient underwent a laboratory evaluation with pulmonary function and exercise tolerance testing.

Pulmonary Function Tests

Tests revealed severe expiratory flow obstruction with marked hyperinflation of static lung volumes (see Table 1). Vital capacity was markedly reduced, and airway resistance was elevated. After bronchodilator administration, there was modest improvement in the expiratory flow rates and vital capacity without much change in the hyperinflated lung volumes. Diffusing capacity was also reduced.

Exercise Study

A two-part exercise test was performed (see Table 2, a and b). The initial test was a maximal, symptom-limited exercise test performed on the treadmill. The patient was able to exercise up to only 0.6 mph and was stopped because of low oxygen saturation. Arterial blood gases demonstrated severe hypoxemia at rest, which worsened with exercise. Analysis of the expired gases showed that there was some minimal remaining ventilatory reserve at the end of this exercise test. V_D/V_T ratio was elevated at rest and with exercise. Anaerobic threshold was not reached. There were no cardiac limitations. Based on the initial study, a steady-state treadmill test was performed with supple-

mental oxygen at 2 L/min. The patient was able to complete 4 minutes of walking at 1.5 mph. Arterial blood gases showed improved oxygenation at rest and during exercise with supplemental oxygen.

Electrocardiogram

Normal sinus rhythm.

Chest Radiograph

Hyperinflation with flattened diaphragm.

Treatment Plan

Based on the initial assessment, the patient was scheduled to begin pulmonary rehabilitation training with the following goals:

- Stabilize pulmonary status at maximum level of function.
- Improve knowledge about lung disease process, condition, and limitations.
- Increase knowledge and understanding of medications, including proper use, effects, and possible side effects.
- Improve muscle strength.
- Reduce dyspnea with use of breathing retraining techniques.
- Improve cough technique.
- Improve ability to pace activities.
- Improve ability to self-assess and report changes in symptoms early to avoid acute care intervention.
- Improve exercise and activity tolerance.
- Improve ability to cope with limitations and panic episodes.
- Improve compliance with continuous oxygen therapy.
- Improve understanding of purpose and use of oxygen therapy.

Pulmonary Rehabilitation Program

Education/Training

The patient attended sessions twice weekly for 4 weeks and weekly for another 4 weeks. Based on the results of the rehabilitation team conference, the patient received training in the following areas:

- Basic lung anatomy and physiology
- Characteristics of COPD and treatment and management of disease

- Breathing retraining exercises
- Controlled cough technique
- Energy-saving techniques
- When to call the doctor
- Oxygen therapy purpose and correct usage
- Nutrition concepts and COPD
- Stress reduction and relaxation
- Concepts in respiratory care, including proper use of MDIs

Exercise

In addition to the training described, the patient began a physical conditioning program to improve exercise tolerance. The exercise prescription included the following:

- Supervised treadmill walks at 1.0 mph for an initial duration of 5 to 10 minutes, with an overall goal of 30 minutes of continuous walking
- A home paced-walking program of 15 steps per 15 seconds (approximately 1.0 mph) for 5 to 10 minutes, increasing the duration as tolerated by breathlessness and muscle fatigue
- Supervised use of an upper body cycle ergometer (UBE) at a level of 200 kpm/min to symptom limit
- A home arm free-weight lifting program with 1-lb weights
- Use of oxygen therapy at 2 L/min continuously

Psychological Support

Group sessions were held weekly with other rehabilitation participants and the team psychologist. Areas discussed included frustration with increasing limitations, depression, public use of oxygen therapy, and panic. Spouses and family members were encouraged to attend.

Summary of Progress

The patient began training at 1.0 mph for 8 minutes with ratings of slight to moderate breathlessness and very little fatigue. Within 1 month exercise tolerance had improved to 30 minutes at the same speed with the patient reporting the same ratings of breathlessness and fatigue.

Compliance with oxygen therapy improved to continuous usage along with a change in belief from "Oxygen not helping" to "It really does help." Use of free weights and the UBE were temporarily discontinued, with the patient being referred to an orthopedist due to discomfort related to a previous shoulder injury.

Through individual discussions and observations, the patient demonstrated an improved ability to use breathing, pacing, and energy-saving techniques. She also demonstrated an improved ability to discuss her disease, symptoms, and treatment. Her confidence improved, and she began doing more. She reported improved performance of activities of daily living as well as a return to some social and recreational activities.

Discharge Plan

A discharge interview was held with the patient to review her progress and encourage her to continue with the exercise and self-care program that she had acquired through rehabilitation training. Her discharge exercise prescription included daily continuous walking at a pace approximating 1.0 mph for 30 minutes. She elected to join a maintenance program for weekly supervised exercise sessions to support her efforts to exercise regularly following discharge from the formal rehabilitation program.

Lung Transplant Evaluation

Shortly after completing the rehabilitation program, the patient and her family began actively investigating lung transplantation programs. She was eventually accepted as a good candidate for single lung transplantation. While she was awaiting surgery, the pulmonary rehabilitation team was consulted for support services with three primary goals: (1) to attain, monitor, and support a maximum level of fitness in this severely impaired patient; (2) to closely monitor symptoms and to report changes early; and (3) to support the patient emotionally during "the wait." Because the surgical date was unknown, the importance of being in shape was stressed.

Pretransplant Rehabilitation

The patient attended the pretransplant program 3 times weekly for 1 hour. She began to train on the treadmill at 1.0 mph for 15 minutes, limited by dyspnea. Chair exercises for upper and lower extremity conditioning were performed at each session. By the 2nd week she had returned to a duration of 30 minutes with only slight breathlessness and fatigue. The patient continued to do well, performing supervised chair exercises and treadmill walks at 30 to 40 minutes at 1.2 mph 3 times weekly, until one visit when she came to the clinic breathless and complaining of a productive cough for 24 to 36 hours and chest discomfort on inspiration. Her physician was notified, and she was taken to the emergency room. Results of the chest X ray confirmed a right lower lobe infiltrate. The patient was admitted and treated with antibiotics. After 6 days she was discharged home.

A few days later she returned to the rehabilitation center complaining of muscle weakness. Her exercise tolerance was decreased to only 7 minutes at a reduced speed of 0.7 mph. Gradually, over a period of 4 weeks, she was able to return to her previous exercise tolerance.

After 5 months, the patient successfully underwent a right single lung transplant.

Posttransplant Hospital Course

Following surgery the patient was mechanically ventilated for 24 hours and was then extubated. She remained in surgical intensive care for 13 days. She was transferred to the floor and remained there for 7 days. She spent 1 week at home, reporting in for clinic appointments with the transplant team.

Posttransplant Rehabilitation

One month after the transplant, the patient returned to the rehabilitation program. At that time she noted a 13-lb weight loss, considerable muscle weakness, and complaints of "feeling shaky" and "fatiguing easily." The patient began a reconditioning program consisting of chair exercises and treadmill walks at 1.0 mph. Initially she was able to walk for only 5 minutes. Oxygen saturations were monitored at each session. Within 2 weeks, the patient's exercise tolerance improved to 30 minutes at 1.25 mph, with oxygen saturations of 94% to 98% on room air. Breathlessness and fatigue were rated as slight. The patient continued training and had increased to 2.0 mph for 30 minutes. She was unable to return to the UBE due to persistent shoulder and elbow discomfort and incisional pain.

In the 7th week post-op, exercise tolerance began to diminish to 15 minutes at 2.0 mph. Ratings of breathlessness and fatigue increased from slight to moderate at a lower level of exercise. Concurrently, the patient began to complain of increased fatigue and a reduced energy level. Oxygen saturations were 96% and unchanged. The patient denied any change in daily monitored peak flow rates. During the rehabilitation session, the patient's physician was notified. After evaluation, the patient was admitted for possible rejection. After 6 days the patient was discharged with the diagnosis of possible cytomegalovirus infection. She continued close follow-up with the transplant team. Eventually she began home intravenous medications for treatment of CMV infection.

After 2 weeks the patient returned to the rehabilitation center, where she resumed training at 1.2 mph on the treadmill for 30 minutes. She continued training and eventually reached a speed of 3.0 mph with a 4% grade for a duration of 30 minutes and denied any breathlessness or fatigue. Three and a half months after returning to the rehabilitation center (4-1/2 months after surgery) the patient graduated from the posttransplant rehabilitation program and joined a health club to begin exercising independently.

Conclusions

Denial of symptoms often delays diagnosis and treatment in COPD patients. This patient was unable to recognize progressive breathlessness until an exacerbation and hospitalization occurred. The patient began to do more and feel better with initial pulmonary rehabilitation training. The patient expressed a renewed sense of hope and self-confidence, which helped her to pursue lung transplantation.

Pretransplant, despite ventilatory limitations, this patient was able to improve exercise tolerance through conditioning training. She was able to sustain an exercise tolerance of 30 minutes' duration until transplantation, except for an acute episode, at which time rehabilitation staff supported early intervention and treatment.

After transplantation, muscle weakness and deconditioning resulting from surgery, weight loss, and inactivity were improved with supervised exercise training from the posttransplant pulmonary rehabilitation program.

Pulmonary rehabilitation is an important component of the pre- and postoperative care of lung transplantation patients.

Table 1 Pulmonary Function Test

Measurement	% Predicted	Prebronchodilator	Postbronchodilator
FVC	28	0.83 L	1.20 L
FEV_1	12	0.27 L	0.38 L
VC	40	1.16 L	1.69 L
TLC	139	6.31 L	6.27 L
RV	309	5.15 L	4.58 L
MIP		50 cm H_2O	. . . .
RAW		10 cm/L	8.0
DLCO	31	6.6 mlco/min/mmHg	. . . .

Table 2a Exercise Study

Rest		Maximum exercise (0.6 mph)	
V_E (L/min BTPS)	10.1	V_E (L/min BTPS)	12.9
ABG: pH	7.43	ABG: pH	7.43
$PaCO_2$	45	$PaCO_2$	44
PaO_2	57	PaO_2	45
O_2 saturation:		O_2 saturation:	
Co-oximeter	90.2%	Co-oximeter	81.2%
Ear oximeter	91%	Ear oximeter	84%
MVV L/min	17	$\dot{V}O_2$ (L/min STPD)	.40
		V_D/V_T (%)	48
		No AT	

Table 2b Oxygen Study

Rest		1.5 mph for 4 min	
O_2	2 L/min	O_2	2 L/min
ABG: pH	7.42	ABG: pH	7.37
$PaCO_2$	44	$PaCO_2$	49
PaO_2	79	PaO_2	63
O_2 saturation:		O_2 saturation:	
Co-oximeter	95.4%	Co-oximeter	90.3%
Ear oximeter	96%	Ear oximeter	92%
		No AT	

Case Study 2

Gerilynn Connors, BS, RRT, RCP

Medical History

L.W. is a 65-year-old man who entered the pulmonary rehabilitation program at discharge from a mental health facility (he had been admitted for depression and suicidal tendencies). L.W. had been diagnosed with emphysema and chronic bronchitis 12 years prior to this visit. He stated that he had noticed a worsening of his condition over the past 2 years. Over the past 2 months he stated that his breathing had deteriorated greatly.

Pulmonary Rehabilitation Team Assessment

Pulmonary Rehabilitation Medical Director

Alert, cooperative, well-developed, and well-nourished man in no acute distress

Heart rate: 104 beats per minute and regular
Blood pressure: 140/98 mmHg
Respiratory rate: 20 breaths per minute with accessory inspiratory muscle use on quiet breathing
Breath sounds: Markedly diminished bilaterally but clear
Heart sounds: Diminished secondary to increased anterior-posterior diameter of chest; no murmur or gallop noted
Liver size: Normal by percussion
Extremities: No clubbing or edema
Medications:
Prednisone: 20 mg with evening meal for the last 2-1/2 years
Xanax: 0.25 mg as needed for nerves
Capoten: 25 mg 3 times a day for hypertension
Ventolin inhaler: 2 puffs a few times a day
No evidence of theophylline nor recollection by patient
Sinequan: 150 mg at bedtime

The following tests are ordered:

- Pre- and postbronchodilator spirometry including DLCO (diffusing capacity), TLC (total lung capacity), and resting ABG (arterial blood gases)
- Posterior/anterior and lateral chest X ray
- PEST (pulmonary exercise stress test)
- Blood chemistry profile
- Assessment by the following team members: nurse, respiratory therapist, physical therapist/occupational therapist, recreation therapist, nutritionist, and psychologist

Respiratory/Nursing Evaluation

L.W. stated he has had a productive cough for the past 20 years and that he wheezes when lying down and with exertion. L.W. has noticed increased shortness of breath (SOB) over the past 2 years, worsening in the last 2 months. Patient was never taught proper breathing techniques and uses accessory muscles on quiet breathing. His breathing pattern is incorrect, with respiratory rate too fast and shallow. Patient uses his inhaler infrequently and incorrectly. L.W. has no knowledge of infection prevention with his lung disease; due to poor understanding of his medications and their usage, he is noncompliant. The following are the results of his pulmonary function test and ABG:

Room air ABG: pH, 7.45; CO_2, 34; O_2, 76; O_2 saturation, 96%
Forced vital capacity (FVC) pre/post: 74%/76% of predicted
Forced expiratory volume in 1 minute (FEV_1) pre/post: 33%/36% of predicted
Forced expiratory flow 25-75 (FEF_{25-75}) pre/post: 10%/11% of predicted
Residual volume (RV): 197% of predicted
DLCO: 25% of predicted

Exercise Evaluation

12-min walk distance: 2,048 feet
MET level: 2.5
O_2 saturation at rest: 93%
O_2 saturation with exercise: 86%

Patient has no current exercise program; poor knowledge of safe exercise guidelines; poor use of diaphragmatic breathing with exercise; low exercise tolerance. PEST showed marked reduction in work capacity with a $\dot{V}O_2$ of 51% of predicted. Anaerobic threshold was reached at 36% of predicted with no breathing reserve, which documents a significant ventilatory limitation to exercise. O_2 saturation dropped to 87% at peak exercise. No ischemic changes were noted on the electrocardiogram, but an occasional premature ventricular contraction was seen during exercise.

Occupational Therapy Evaluation

Activities of daily living produce SOB during showering and drying off, which make it difficult for the patient and produce fear of taking a shower. SOB occurs while dressing, reaching, bending, and personal grooming. The patient lives on the second floor, and stairs present a barrier. Patient tires easily and is withdrawn and seclusive.

Psychosocial Evaluation

Patient is frustrated and fearful over his worsening SOB. With recent hospital admission to the mental health unit for depression and suicidal tendencies, the patient has become concerned about functioning in society. Patient will continue with psychiatric treatment during the pulmonary program. Patient feels useless due to his lung disease.

Nutritional Evaluation

Patient is about 15 lb underweight with his current weight at 127-1/2 lb (target weight is 140-148 lb). Patient's lipid profile is as follows:

Total cholesterol: 227 mg/dL
High density lipoproteins: 60 mg/dL
Low density lipoproteins: 148 mg/dL
Risk ratio: 3.8

Patient claims he has lost weight in the last 3 months despite eating well. Patient had an ulcer in 1983 and reports no current problems. Percent body fat is 19.4.

Recreational Therapy Evaluation

Patient states he has lost his desire to live. He feels that his chronic obstructive pulmonary disease is trapping him. He does not like getting out and socializing and has no motivation. Patient is having difficulty in self-care tasks, including a fear of showering. Patient reports SOB while dressing, reaching, and bending. Patient is retired and as a result has an abundance of leisure time but is not motivated to do much. Patient does have a flight of stairs to maneuver at home, and they present a barrier to him. Patient is SOB and unable to relax during the interview. Patient tires easily and panics, thereby losing control of his breathing.

Other Diagnostic Test Results

Blood chemistry panel including thyroid function tests:

T4 elevated: 14.9 mcg/dL
(normal 4.7-12.7)
T7 (FTI): 5.7 mcg/dL
(normal 1.8 to 4.4)

A thyroid scan demonstrated an increased uptake diffusely. The patient was diagnosed with hyperthyroidism. Many of his complaints, including emotional instability, rapid heart rate, hand tremors, weakness, and worsening of SOB, could be related to the presence of thyrotoxicosis. Patient is being referred to an endocrinologist for evaluation and treatment of his hyperthyroidism.

Diagnosis

Chronic bronchitis, emphysema, hyperthyroidism, cushionoid side effects related to exogenous prednisone, hypertension, history of peptic ulcer, depression, heartburn, and postnasal drainage

Treatment Plan/Pulmonary Rehabilitation Program

Patient to participate in a 5-week outpatient pulmonary rehabilitation program. The program is to address the target areas determined during the initial team evaluations.

The following areas were addressed during the pulmonary rehabilitation program based upon the initial assessment:

- Proper diaphragmatic breathing with pursed-lip breathing
- Proper utilization of metered-dose inhaler
- Adequate understanding of oral medication regimen, resulting in appropriate compliance
- Maintenance and reinforcement of smoking cessation
- Training related to environmental factors affecting symptoms
- Training in and understanding of lung structure and function
- Training in and understanding of exercise guidelines

- Structured daily exercise program
- Breathing retraining with pursed-lip breathing and diaphragmatic breathing
- Improvement in body posture
- Increased exercise tolerance through an exercise training program, 1 hour each day, 3 days a week for 5 weeks
- Dietary intervention to reduce body fat to 15%
- Dietary weight gain program while on a low-fat diet; nutritional supplements for weight gain
- Energy conservation and work simplification skills
- Proper breathing with exercise
- Increased upper extremity strength
- Increased and improved socialization
- Reduced feelings of depression
- Principles of balance in life tasks
- Increased knowledge and resources for leisure activities
- Training on nutrition and lung disease

Discharge Home Recommendations

After completing the 5-week program, the patient was advised to adhere to the following recommendations at home:

- Practice pursed-lip with diaphragmatic breathing 5 minutes twice a day in standing, sitting and lying positions, with 8- to 12-lb weights while in lying position.
- Use Aerochamber with inhaler.
- Do home exercise program to consist of warm-up, aerobic exercise at a target heart rate of 20 to 22 beats in 10 seconds (126 beats per minute), and cool-down. Exercise should be done 20 minutes at least 4 to 6 times per week working to a total exercise time of 30 minutes. Pulse taken at wrist or neck.
- Do exercise program of walking or stationary cycling by intervals on "bad days" (when breathing is worse) following any row of the chart from start to finish:

Exercise	Rest	Exercise	Rest	Exercise
2 min	1 min	2 min	1 min	2 min
5	2	5	2	2
10	2	5	2	5
15	2	10	2	5

- Practice stress reduction exercise (autogenic relaxation exercise or visualization for health and relaxation) 15 to 20 minutes daily.
- Use social structure for stress management.
- Increase awareness of early signs of physical and emotional stress.
- Plan your day to include something that makes you smile or feel good about yourself.
- Incorporate energy conservation/work simplification techniques into activities of daily living.
- Use panic control techniques when short of breath.
- Do upper extremity strengthening exercises with proper breathing (see handouts for recommended exercises).
- Achieve 15-lb weight gain (current weight: 127-1/2 lb; target weight: 140-148 lb). Follow a low-fat, high-complex carbohydrate diet; choose whole grains, vegetables, and fruit. Reduce or omit intake of fatty meats, cheeses, eggs, oils, dressings, butter or margarine, and rich desserts. Limit sugar intake. Use extra fat, preferably in the form of nuts, avocado, or some vegetable oils, to assist with your weight-gain program.
- Keep properly hydrated: drink 8 to 10 glasses of water a day, 10 to 12 glasses if the weather is hot, your temperature is elevated, or you have an infection.
- Review the pulmonary rehabilitation training manual at least once a week and share information with your family and friends.
- Have a (once-in-a-lifetime) pneumococcal vaccine.
- Get a flu shot every year in September or October.
- Continue to work on smoking cessation.

The patient was advised to use these medications in the specified doses:

Theodur: 300-mg tab; 1 tab twice a day
Capoten: 25-mg tab; 1 tab 3 times a day
Nasalide nasal spray: 2 sprays in each nostril twice a day
Zantac: 150-mg tab; 1 tab at bedtime, and 1 tab twice a day if needed to control stomach pain
Sinequan: 75-mg capsule; 1 capsule at bedtime
Prednisone: 5-mg tabs; tapering schedule in the following sequence:
12.5 mg every morning × 5 days
10 mg every morning × 5 days

7.5 mg every morning × 5 days
5 mg every morning × 5 days
10 mg every other day for 6 days
7.5 mg every other day for 6 days
5 mg every other day for 6 days
2.5 mg every other day for 6 days
Stop taking prednisone.

    If at any time during the tapering schedule patient notices worsening of breathing with increasing cough or shortness of breath, he is to return to the next larger dosage of prednisone at which he was stable. He is to stay at this level for 1 week, and then try again to taper, according to the same schedule.

Ventolin inhaler: 2 puffs 4 times a day, up to 6 times a day; patient to use Aerochamber with inhaler

Vanceril inhaler: 2 puffs 4 times a day, 10 minutes after Ventolin inhaler; patient to use Aerochamber with inhaler

Mylanta 2: About 2 tablespoons at bedtime as needed for upset stomach

Augmentin: 250-mg tabs; 1 tab 3 times a day for 7 days for respiratory infection; patient to keep a supply of this antibiotic at home

Patient should check theophylline level after thyroid treatment to verify that current dose of theophylline is sufficient.

If the patient remains symptom-free by using 1 Zantac pill at bedtime, he may try stopping Zantac altogether. If he still remains symptom-free, he need no longer take Zantac.

Oxygen is not necessary for the patient to fly in a commercial airliner. Flying to Hawaii will be safe for him only after treatment for his thyroid condition.

Patient is being referred to an ear-nose-throat specialist for evaluation.

Patient is seeing an endocrinologist for evaluation and treatment of his thyroid condition.

Records to be sent to the patient's primary doctor and the patient.

Summary

The patient completed the 5-week program with improvement in his symptoms of dypsnea and depression. He successfully continued his rehabilitation at home. The patient returned to his primary care physician for follow-up and has continued to be re-evaluated by the rehabilitation team yearly. Through program compliance, the patient has improved his overall quality of life and exercise tolerance.

List of Training Resources

A special thank-you to Beverly Striplin, a volunteer and graduate of the pulmonary rehabilitation program at Mt. Diablo Medical Center, for assisting in the editing of Appendix D.

Appendix current as of July 1, 1992. For additional resources contact your local or national home medical equipment supplier, pharmaceutical company, or the American Lung Association.

A.V. Equipment

Key:
AARC = American Association for Respiratory Care
ALA = American Lung Association
BO = Booklet
S/T = Slides and audiotape
Tape = Audiotape
VHS = Videotape

Title	Type	Company	Address/phone
The Asthma Handbook	S/T & BO	ALA	1740 Broadway New York, NY 10019 (212) 315-8700
Be in Control of Your Lungs (Patient Discharge Teaching)	Tape/BO	Gretchen Peske, Pulmonary Re-habilitation Ed.	3135 Attleboro Place Greensburg, PA 15601 (412) 836-5359
Benefits of Pulmonary Rehab	VHS	Lifestyle & Behavioral Management	2720 Lamont Rd. Louisville, KY 40205 (502) 459-7324
Better Breathing Today	Tape/BO	Health Communica-tion Services, Inc.	249 S. Highway 101, Ste. 434 Solano Beach, CA 92075 (619) 755-2459
Better Breathing, Better Living	VHS	Vermont Lung Assoc.	30 Farrel St. S. Burlington, VT 05403 (802) 863-6817
Better Breathers Panic Control Workbook	Tape/Book	California College for Health Sciences	222 W. 24th St. National City, CA 91950 (800) 221-7374
Beyond Stress Series: *Breathing Away Stress* *Relaxing Muscle Tension* *The Relaxation Response* *Focusing the Mind* *Maximizing Performance* *The Session*	VHS	TVO Video	1140 Kildaire Farm Rd. Cary, NC 27511 (800) 331-9566
Be Your Own Pacemaker (Relaxation tape)	Tape	Lifestyle & Behavioral Management	2720 Lamont Rd. Louisville, KY 40205 (502) 459-7324
A Breath of Life: Pulmonary Rehabilitation	VHS	UCSD Medical Center, Pulmonary Rehabilita-tion Program	225 Dickinson St. (H-772) San Diego, CA 92103-1990 (619) 294-6066
Bronchial Asthma	VHS	Milner Fenwick, Inc.	2125 Greenspring Dr. Timonium, MD 21093 (410) 252-1700
Clearing Your Airways	VHS	Appleton & Lange Media	25 Van Zant St. East Norwalk, CT 06855 (800) 826-2618
Chairobics—Home Pulmonary Rehab	VHS	Chairobics—Home Pulmonary Rehab	(800) 521-7303

(continued)

Title	Type	Company	Address/phone
Choices—The Key Is You	VHS	Health Communication Services, Inc.	249 S. Highway 101, Ste. 434 Solano Beach, CA 92075 (619) 755-2459
Daydreams	Tape	Whole Person Assoc.	1702 E. Jefferson St. P.O. Box 3151 Duluth, MN 55812 (800) 247-6789
Death in the West	VHS	Pyramid Film and Video	P.O. Box 1048 Santa Monica, CA 90406-1048 (800) 421-2304
Do You Really Know How to Breathe?	VHS	Pal Medical, Inc.	235 S. Maitland Ave., Ste. 214 Maitland, FL 32751 (407) 298-8083
Eating Well With Pulmonary Disease	VHS	Ross Laboratories	625 Cleveland Ave. Columbus, OH 43215 (614) 227-3583
Fat Stuff	VHS	MTI Film & Video	920 Academy Dr. Northbrook, IL 60062 (800) 621-2131
The Feminine Mistake: The Next Generation	VHS	Pyramid Film and Video	P.O. Box 1048 Santa Monica, CA 90406-1048 (800) 421-2304
Help Yourself to Better Breathing	VHS	ALA	1740 Broadway New York, NY 10019 (212) 315-8700
How to Beat Cigarettes	VHS	Milner Fenwick, Inc.	2125 Greenspring Timonium, MD 21093 (410) 252-1700
How to Use Your Attachment Devices for MDI	VHS	Allen & Hanburys Division of Glaxo	Contact your local pharmaceutical representative.
How to Use Your Pulmo-Aid Compressor	VHS	DiVilbiss Health Care, Inc.	1200 East Main Street Somerset, PA 15501-0635 (814) 443-4881
How to Use Your Ventolin Rotohaler	VHS	Allen & Hanburys Division of Glaxo	Contact your local pharmaceutical representative.
How You Can Help Patients Stop Smoking: Opportunities for Respiratory Care Practitioners	VHS/BO	AARC	11030 Ables Lane Dallas, TX 75229 (214) 243-2272
I Am Joe's Lung: New Version	VHS	Pyramid Film and Video	P.O. Box 1048 Santa Monica, CA 90406-1048 (800) 421-2304
I Am Joe's Heart: New Version	VHS	Pyramid Film and Video	P.O. Box 1048 Santa Monica, CA 90406-1048 (800) 421-2304
Is It Worth Dying For? (Stress)	VHS	Medical Research	4600 S. Ulster St., Ste. 700 Denver, CO 80237 (303) 694-0647

Title	Type	Company	Address/phone

Living With Emphysema
Five Part Series
  1. *Development and Detection*
  2. *Diagnosis*
  3. *Treatment*
  4. *Rehabilitation*
  5. *Family Support*
	VHS	Aims Media	9710 DeSoto Ave.
			Chatsworth, CA 91311
			(800) 367-2467

Living With Stress	VHS	Milner Fenwick, Inc.	2125 Greenspring Dr. Timonium, MD 21093 (410) 252-1700
Making A Difference, Opportunities for *Smoking Cessation Counseling*	VHS	National Heart, Lung, and Blood Institute (NHLBI), Smoking Education Program	P.O. Box 30105 Bethesda, MD 20824-0105 (301) 951-3260
Maintaining Intimacy for the Short of *Breath*	Tape/Book	California College for Health Sciences	222 W. 24th St. National City, CA 91950 (800) 221-7374
Medications Working for You	S/T	ALA of Orange County	1570 E. 17th St. Santa Ana, CA 92701 (714) 835-5864
Metered Dose Inhaler Techniques	VHS	Allen & Hanburys Division of Glaxo	Contact your local pharma- ceutical representative.
The Missing Piece	VHS	Patient to Patient, Inc.	450 Main St. Port Jefferson, NY 11777 (516) 928-9000
Nicotine Intervention Kit	VHS	AARC	11030 Ables Lane Dallas, TX 75229 (214) 243-2272
The Normal Lung and COPD	VHS	Appleton & Lange Media	25 Van Zant St. East Norwalk, CT 06855 (800) 826-2618
Nutrition for Better Health	VHS	Milner Fenwick, Inc.	2125 Greenspring Dr. Timonium, MD 21093 (410) 252-1700
Overview of Allergies	VHS	Allen & Hanburys Division of Glaxo	Contact your local pharma- ceutical representative.
Overview of Asthma	VHS	Allen & Hanburys Division of Glaxo	Contact your local pharma- ceutical representative.

PEP Series
  How the Lungs Work
  What is COPD?
  Chronic Bronchitis
  What is Emphysema?
  Understanding Asthma
  Drug Therapy of COPD
  Inhalation Therapy
  Oxygen Therapy
  Breathing Exercises
  General Health Measures
	VHS & S/T	ALA of Georgia	2452 Spring Road
			Smyrna, GA 30080
			(404) 434-5864

(continued)

Title	Type	Company	Address/phone
Pulmonary Rehabilitation	VHS	AARC	11030 Ables Lane Dallas, TX 75229 (214) 243-2272

Pulmonary Self-Care
4-part Series:
    Living With a Breathing Problem
    Learning to Breathe Better
    Clearing Our Airways
    Building Your Strength and Endurance
	VHS	Training Edge, Inc.	502 N. Plum Grove Rd.
			Palatine, IL 60067
			(800) 292-4375

Relaxation Techniques for Better Breathing	Tape	California College for Health Sciences	222 W. 24th St. National City, CA 91950 (800) 221-7374
Scenes: Coping With COPD	VHS	Vermont Lung Assoc.	30 Farrel St. S. Burlington, VT 05403 (802) 863-6817
Secondhand Smoke	VHS	Pyramid Film and Video	P.O. Box 1048 Santa Monica, CA 90406-1048 (800) 421-2304

Self-Help: Your Strategy for Living with COPD
    1. COPD: What Is It?
    2. Learning Helpful Ways to Breathe
    3. Clearing Your Lungs to Help You
        Breathe Easier, Parts 1 & 2
	VHS/BO	Bull Publishing Co.	P.O. Box 208
			Palo Alto, CA 94302
			(800) 676-2855

Sexual Counseling Series:
For the M.D.
    A Visit With Harry
    A Visit With Helen
	S/T	Pulmonary Foundation	1011 Ruth St.
			Prescott, AZ 86301
			(602) 445-6025

Smoking: Everything You and Your Family Need to Know	VHS	Ambrose Video Publishing	1290 Avenue of the Americas New York, NY 10104 (800) 526-4663
So You Have Asthma, Too!	VHS	Allen & Hanburys Division of Glaxo	Contact your local pharmaceutical representative.

St. John's Hospital Series
    Breathing Easier
    Chronic Lung Disease
    Living With It: Asthma
	VHS	St. John's Hospital	c/o Care Video Productions
			P.O. Box 45132
			Cleveland, OH 44145
			(216) 835-5872

Stress and COPD	VHS	Appleton & Lange Media	25 Van Zant St. East Norwalk, CT 06855 (800) 826-2618

Stress Management Series
    Stressbreak
    Relaxation
    Relaxation—Changing Behavior
    Healing Journey
    Rainbow Butterfly
	VHS
	VHS
	VHS
	VHS
	Tape
	Tape
		Source Cassette Learning Systems	(800) 52TAPES

Take a Deep Breath With Terry Bradshaw	VHS	Shumpert Medical Center, Pulmonary Rehabilitation	915 Margaret Pl. Shreveport, LA 71101 (318) 227-6645

Title	Type	Company	Address/phone
Tips for Living With COPD	VHS	Appleton and Lange Media	25 Van Zant St. East Norwalk, CT 06855 (800) 826-2618
A Touch in the Night	Tape	California College for Health Sciences	222 W. 24th St. National City, CA 91950 (800) 221-7374
Tracheostomy Care	VHS	ALA of Oklahoma	P.O. Box 53303 Oklahoma City, OK 73152 (405) 524-8471
Traveling With Lung Disease (by Dr. Joel Seidman)	VHS	Medical Center of Central Massachusetts Memorial, Pulmonary Rehabilitation	119 Belmont St. Worcester, MA 01605 (508) 793-6637
Understanding Allergies	VHS	Milner Fenwick, Inc.	2125 Greenspring Dr. Timonium, MD 21093 (410) 252-1700
Your Lungs, The Tree of Life (How to Use Azmacort Inhaler)	VHS	Rorer Pharmaceuticals Corporation	500 Arcola Rd. Collegeville, PA 19426 (215) 628-6000

Brochures/Booklets

Key:
AARC = American Association for Respiratory Care
ALA = American Lung Association
BO = Booklet
BR = Brochure
DI = Directory

Title	Type	Company	Address/phone
AAT Deficiency and Your Lungs	BO	Miles, Inc. Pharmaceutical Division, Biological Products	545 Long Wharf New Haven, CT 06511 (203) 937-2000
AAT Deficiency and Your Patients— A Guide for Nurses	BO	Miles, Inc. Pharmaceutical Division, Biological Products	545 Long Wharf New Haven, CT 06511 (203) 937-2000
The ABCs of Smoking	BR	Health Edco Division of WRS Group	P.O. Box 21207 Waco, TX 76702-1207 (800) 299-3366
About Emphysema	BO	Channing L. Bete Co., Inc.	200 State Rd. S. Deerfield, MA 01373 (800) 628-7733
Action Guide on Smoking	BR	Health Edco Division of WRS Group	P.O. Box 21207 Waco, TX 76702-1207 (800) 299-3366
To Air is Human	BO	Pritchett & Hull Assoc., Inc.	3440 Oakcliff Rd., NE, Ste. 110 Atlanta, GA 30340 (800) 241-4925
Around the Clock With COPD (Energy Conservation Booklet)	BO	ALA	1740 Broadway New York, NY 10019 (212) 315-8700 Or your local office
Asthma	BR	AARC	11030 Ables Ln. Dallas, TX 75229 (214) 243-2272
The Asthma Attack	BR	Milner Fenwick, Inc.	2125 Greenspring Dr. Timonium, MD 21093 (410) 252-1700
Asthma—The New Way of Life	BR	Milner Fenwick, Inc.	2125 Greenspring Dr. Timonium, MD 21093 (410) 252-1700
Asthma: Treatment	BR	Milner Fenwick, Inc.	2125 Greenspring Dr. Timonium, MD 21093 (410) 252-1700
Becoming Close	BO	National Jewish Center for Immunology and Respiratory Medicine	1400 Jackson St. Denver, CO 80206 (800) 222-LUNG
Black Lung	BO	National Jewish Center for Immunology and Respiratory Medicine	1400 Jackson St. Denver, CO 80206 (800) 222-LUNG
Brief Guide to Home Care Services for Those With Lung Problems	BO	ALA of New York	8 Mountain View Ave. Albany, NY 12205 (914) 459-4197

Title	Type	Company	Address/phone
Bronchitis	BR	Ninco	P.O. Box 9 Calhoun, KY 42327 (800) 962-6662
Calling It Quits	BR	ALA	1740 Broadway New York, NY 10019 (212) 315-8700 Or your local office
Coping With Indoor Air Pollution	BR	AARC	11030 Ables Ln. Dallas, TX 75229 (214) 243-2272
Dealing With Allergies	BR	AARC	11030 Ables Ln. Dallas, TX 75229 (214) 243-2272
Eating Right: Tips for the COPD Patient	BR	AARC	11030 Ables Ln. Dallas, TX 75229 (214) 243-2272
Emphysema	BR	Ninco	P.O. Box 9 Calhoun, KY 42327 (800) 962-6662
The Essentials of Pulmonary Rehabilitation Parts I and II	BO	Thomas Petty, MD	1719 East 19th Ave. Denver, CO 80218 (303) 939-6740
Eurolung Assistance	DI	F. Smeets, MD	Centre Hospitalier de Sainte-Ode 6680 Sainte Ode Tenneville, Belgium (32) 084-45-54-44
Exercising Safely With COPD	BR	AARC	11030 Ables Ln. Dallas, TX 75229 (214) 243-2272
Facts About Asthma	BR	ALA	1740 Broadway New York, NY 10019 (212) 315-8700 Or your local office
Facts About Lungs and Lung Disease	BR	ALA	1740 Broadway New York, NY 10019 (212) 315-8700 Or your local office
Freedom From Smoking	BO	ALA	1740 Broadway New York, NY 10019 (212) 315-8700 Or your local office
Helping Your Child Breathe Easier	BR	AARC	11030 Ables Ln. Dallas, TX 75229 (214) 243-2272
How to Stop Smoking	BO	Channing L. Bete Co., Inc.	200 State Rd. S. Deerfield, MA 01373 (800) 628-7733
How You Can Help Patients Stop Smoking: Opportunities for Respiratory Care Practitioners	BO	National Heart, Lung, and Blood Institute (NHLBI), Smoking Education Program	P.O. Box 30105 Bethesda, MD 20824-0105 (301) 951-3260

(continued)

Title	Type	Company	Address/phone
Indoor Air Pollution	BR	AARC	11030 Ables Ln. Dallas, TX 75229 (214) 243-2272
If You Smoke—Here's What Your Doctor May See	BR	Health Connection Narcotics Education, Inc.	55 Oak Ridge Dr. Hagerstown, MD 21740 (800) 548-8700
Lessening the Effects of COPD	BR	AARC	11030 Ables Ln. Dallas, TX 75229 (214) 243-2272
Living With Asthma	BR	AARC	11030 Ables Ln. Dallas, TX 75229 (214) 243-2272
Making a Choice About Smoking	BO	Channing L. Bete Co., Inc.	200 State Rd. S. Deerfield, MA 01373 (800) 628-7733
Minimizing the Effects of Outdoor Air Pollution	BR	AARC	11030 Ables Ln. Dallas, TX 75229 (214) 243-2272
A New Wrinkle Smoking Program	BR	Health Connection Narcotics Education, Inc.	55 Oak Ridge Dr. Hagerstown, MD 21740 (800) 548-8700
Nicotine Dependency Program How You Can Help Patients Stop Smoking	BO	AARC	11030 Ables Ln. Dallas, TX 75229 (214) 243-2272
A Patient's Guide to Asthma	BO	Allen & Hansburys Division of Glaxo	Contact your local pharmaceutical representative.
Prolastin, Alpha$_1$-Proteinase Inhibitor (Human): Answers To Important Questions About Safety	BO	Miles, Inc. Pharmaceutical Division, Biological Products	545 Long Wharf New Haven, CT 06511 (203) 937-2000
Prolastin, Alpha$_1$-Proteinase Inhibitor (Human): Product Monograph	BO	Miles, Inc. Pharmaceutical Division, Biological Products	545 Long Wharf New Haven, CT 06511 (203) 937-2000
The Process of Quitting Smoking	BR	AARC	11030 Ables Ln. Dallas, TX 75229 (214) 243-2272
Quitting for Life	BR	Health Edco, Division of WRS Group	P.O. Box 21207 Waco, TX 76702-1207 (800) 299-3366
Requirements for Traveling With Oxygen	BO	AARC	11030 Ables Ln. Dallas, TX 75229 (214) 243-2272
Respiratory Allergies	BR	AARC	11030 Ables Ln. Dallas, TX 75229 (214) 243-2272
Secondhand Smoke	BR	AARC	11030 Ables Ln. Dallas, TX 75229 (214) 243-2272

Title	Type	Company	Address/phone
Self-Help: Your Strategy for Living With COPD	BO	Bull Publishing Co.	P.O. Box 208 Palo Alto, CA 94302 (415) 322-2855
Simplicity—The Key to Therapy for Congenital Emphysema	BO	Miles, Inc. Pharmaceutical Division, Biological Products	545 Long Wharf New Haven, CT 06511 (203) 937-2000
Smokeless Tobacco	BR	Health Edco, Division of WRS Group	P.O. Box 21207 Waco, TX 76702-1207 (800) 299-3366
Smoking and Your Heart	BO	Channing L. Bete Co., Inc.	200 State Rd. S. Deerfield, MA 01373 (800) 628-7733
Starving for Air: What Emphysema May Do	BR	Health Connection Narcotics Education, Inc.	55 Oak Ridge Dr. Hagerstow, MD 21740 (800) 548-8700
Your Guide to Controlling Cholesterol	BO	Health Trend Publications	P.O. Box 17420-A Encino, CA 91416-7420 (818) 906-7120

Title	Type	Company	Address/phone
Air Currents	Newsletter	Allen & Hanburys Division of Glaxo	Contact your local pharmaceutical representative.
Airlines	Newsletter	ALA of New Hampshire	456 Beech St., Box 1014 Manchester, NH 03105 (603) 669-2411
Air Line	Newsletter	ALA of Atlanta	723 Piedmont Ave., NE Atlanta, GA 30365 (404) 872-9653
Airways	Newsletter	ALA of SE Michigan	18860 W. 10 Mile Rd. Southfield, MI 48075 (313) 559-5100
Alpha 1 News	Newsletter	Peter Smith	819 Bayview Rd. Neenah, WI 54956 (414) 725-7046
Asthma Resources Directory	Book	Allergy Publications Inc.	P.O. Box 640 Menlo Park, CA 94026-0640
Batting the Breeze	Newsletter	Emphysema Anonymous, Inc.	P.O. Box 3224 Seminole, FL 34642 (813) 391-9977
Chek-Med Card	Drug cards	Chek-Med Systems	75 Utley Dr. Camp Hill, PA 17011 (800) 848-2891
Cholesterol Control Made Easy	Book	Health Trend Publications	P.O. Box 17420-A Encino, CA 91416-7420 (818) 906-7120
Enjoying Life With Emphysema	Book	Thomas Petty, MD	Williams & Wilkins Attn: Editorial Department 428 East Preston St. Baltimore, MD 21202 (800) 638-0672
Heartbeat	Book	Health Trend Publications	P.O. Box 17420-A Encino, CA 91416-7420 (818) 906-7120
Living Well With Emphysema and Bronchitis	Book	Doubleday & Co.	666 E. Fifth Ave. New York, NY 10103 (800) 223-6834
"Lung Line"	Phoneline	National Jewish Center for Immunology and Respiratory Medicine	1400 Jackson St. Denver, CO 80206 (303) 388-4461
Mainstay	Book	ALA of the San Jacinto Area	3100 Weslayan, No. 330 Houston, TX 77027 (713) 968-5800
The MA Report	Newsletter	Mothers of Asthmatics	10875 Main St., Ste. 210 Fairfax, VA 22030 (703) 385-4403
New Trends in Asthma, General Information	Newsletter	Allen & Hanburys Division of Glaxo	Contact your local pharmaceutical representative.

Title	Type	Company	Address/phone
A Patient's Guide to Asthma	Book	Allen & Hanburys Division of Glaxo	Contact your local pharmaceutical representative.
The Pulmonary Paper	Newsletter	Celeste Belyea	P.O. Box 217 Exeter, NH 03833
Second Wind Newsletter	Newsletter	Little Company of Mary Hospital	4101 Torrance Blvd. Torrance, CA 90503 (310) 543-5979
Shortness of Breath ''A Guide to Better Living and Breathing'' (3rd edition)	Book	CV Mosby Co.	11830 Westline Industrial Dr. St. Louis, MO 63146 (314) 872-8370
Teaching Manuals *Air Power* *Living With Asthma* *Airwise* *Open Airways-Respiro Abierto*	 Manual Manual Manual Manual	National Heart, Lung, & Blood Institute (NHLBI), Asthma Project	P.O. Box 30105 Bethesda, MD 20824-0105 (301) 951-3260

Index

Entries from tables and figures are identified in italics.

About the AACVPR

Statement of Purpose

Recognizing that cardiovascular and pulmonary rehabilitation is a multidisciplinary field, the American Association of Cardiovascular and Pulmonary Rehabilitation (AACVPR) is dedicated to the improvement of clinical practice, promotion of scientific inquiry, and advancement of education for the benefit of the health-care professional and the public.

Objectives

The AACVPR strives to

- provide professional education through sponsorship and/or promotion of educational conferences, scientific meetings, and publications;
- provide a forum for information exchange through a resource center that proactively communicates with health-care professionals to effect delivery of quality health-care services;
- encourage, coordinate, and/or sponsor research that will enhance understandings of rehabilitation impact on disease processes, the health and personal welfare of patients, and the social health-care support systems;
- promote throughout the public sector understandings as to the nature of rehabilitation and increase awareness of the related health-care services available across the nation;
- cooperate and/or collaborate with other organizations having interests similar to those of the Association;
- provide ways and means to enhance career development for Association members.

Membership Benefits

- Receive the *Journal of Cardiopulmonary Rehabilitation* monthly, keeping you updated on current research and information in the field of rehabilitation.
- Be part of a national network of professionals dedicated to the advancement of cardiovascular and pulmonary rehabilitation.
- Receive a quarterly newsletter containing information about practical issues.
- Have the opportunity to attend regional seminars and the AACVPR Annual Meeting.
- Be included in and have access to the national membership directory and national program directory.
- Be a part of a great networking system and have access to nationwide job opportunities.
- Receive up-to-date information on federal and state guidelines, reimbursement for rehabilitation services, and other issues of concern to professionals in the field.
- Have the opportunity to publish articles in the *Journal of Cardiopulmonary Rehabilitation* and present original research at the Annual Meeting.

We invite you to meet the challenge and become involved in the AACVPR. Decide to join this dynamic organization today. Fill out the membership application included in this book and send it to the AACVPR. The professional growth that you will experience by becoming a member of this Association will benefit you for years to come. We look forward to your future support and contributions.

American Association of Cardiovascular and Pulmonary Rehabilitation

MEMBERSHIP APPLICATION

Name _____ Male ☐ Female ☐ _____/_____/_____
Birthdate

Mailing address _____
Office or clinic
_____
Street
_____ _____
City   State   Zip/postal code
_____ ( )_____/( )_____
Country   Telephone   /Fax

CURRENT PROGRAM INVOLVEMENT (Check all that apply)

Job title: _____

☐ Cardiovascular rehabilitation   ☐ Pulmonary rehabilitation   ☐ State Society Member   Where did you hear about AACVPR?
    ☐ Inpatient   ☐ Inpatient   ☐ work   ☐ JCR
    ☐ Outpatient   ☐ Outpatient   ☐ other member   ☐ professional colleague
☐ Other (specify): _____   ☐ school/university   ☐ other

MEMBERSHIP CATEGORIES

Select and complete only one category. Requirements are listed on the back of this application.

MEMBER				
☐ **Physician**	☐ **Scientist**	☐ **Allied health**	☐ **Educator**	☐ **Nurse**
☐ Cardiology ☐ Pulmonary ☐ Internal medicine ☐ Family/general practice ☐ Other	•Degree(s): _____ •Principle field of education: _____ •Certification/licensure: _____	•Degree(s): _____ •Principle field of education: _____ •Certification/licensure: _____	•Degree(s): _____ •Principle field of education: _____ •Certification/licensure: _____	•Degree(s): _____ •Certification/licensure: _____
_____ $120.00 per year	$120.00 per year	$120.00 per year	$120.00 per year	$120.00 per year

☐ **STUDENT MEMBER**

Institution: _____

Major: _____

Full-time credit load at your institution: _____

Number of credits you are currently taking: _____

Year degree expected: _____
                 month   year
$60.00 per year

☐ **ASSOCIATE MEMBER**

Primary occupation: _____

Institution: _____

Major area(s) of interest: _____

_____
$120.00 per year

I certify that the above information is correct, and I agree to abide by the Code of Ethics and Professional Conduct of the American Association of Cardiovascular and Pulmonary Rehabilitation.

_____ _____
Signature   Date

Mail application with check or money order in
U.S. currency to: **AACVPR**
                7611 Elmwood Avenue, Suite 201
                Middleton, WI 53562
                608-831-6989

Where did you hear about the AACVPR?

_____

_____

Code of Ethical and Professional Conduct

A. Objectives
This code is designed to aid the Fellows and Members of the Association, individually and collectively, to maintain a high level of ethical and professional conduct. The code may be considered a standard by which a Fellow or Member may determine the propriety of his or her conduct and relationship with colleagues, members of allied professions, the public, and all persons with whom a professional relationship has been established. These should be concordant with the principal purpose of the Association, which is the improvement of clinical practice, promotion of scientific inquiry, and advancement of education for the benefit of health-care professionals and the public in the multidisciplinary field of cardiovascular and pulmonary rehabilitation.

Fellows and Members should strive continuously to improve their knowledge and skills and to make available to their colleagues and to the public the benefits of their professional attainments.

Fellows and Members should maintain high professional and scientific standards and should not voluntarily associate professionally with those who violate this principle.

The Association should safeguard the public and itself against Fellows or Members who are deficient in ethical conduct or professional competence.

B. Maintenance of Good Standing in Regulated Professions
Any Fellow or Member required by law to be licensed, certified, or otherwise regulated by any government agency or professional association in order to practice his or her profession must remain in good standing before that agency or association as a condition of continued membership in the American Association of Cardiovascular and Pulmonary Rehabilitation. Any expulsion, suspension, probation, or other sanction imposed by such government or professional body on any Fellow or Member may be grounds for disciplinary action by the Association.

C. Public Disclosure of Affiliation
Any Fellow or Member may make disclosure of affiliation with the Association in an appropriate professional context, including use in curriculum vitae, in biographical descriptions, or in another professional, dignified manner. Disclosure of affiliation may not be made in connection with any commercial venture without prior written authorization of the Association. A commercial venture is defined here to mean the sale of any goods, services, or other property for a valuable consideration with the exception of books, journal articles, or other professional publications. Requests for such authorization should be made in writing to the President or the Executive Director of the Association. Fellows may list their affiliation with the Association on professional or business cards, only by the use of the initials F.A.A.C.V.P.R.; members other than Fellows may not use this affiliation on business or professional cards. Disclosure in violation of these guidelines may be grounds for disciplinary action.

The use of the name of the American Association of Cardiovascular and Pulmonary Rehabilitation as a cosponsoring or cooperating organization for professional meetings, professional education programs, and the like must follow the guidelines of the Association for these specific designations.

D. Discipline
Any Fellow or Member of the Association may be disciplined or expelled for conduct which, in the opinion of the Board of Directors, is derogatory to the dignity or inconsistent with the purposes of the Association. The expulsion of a Fellow or Member may be ordered upon the affirmative vote of two-thirds of the members of the Board of Directors present at a regular or special meeting and only after such Fellow or Member has been informed of the charges preferred and has been given an opportunity to refute such charges before the Board of Directors. Other disciplinary action such as reprimand, probation, or censure may be recommended by the Committee on Ethics and Professional Conduct and ordered following the affirmative vote of at least two-thirds of the members of the Board of Directors present at a regular or special meeting or by mail ballot, provided a quorum take action.

Membership Requirements

Member
Shall be any interested person of majority age who is a physician, medical scientist, allied health-care practitioner, or educator, and who in his or her professional endeavors, is regularly involved in some aspect of cardiovascular and/or pulmonary rehabilitation. Members have AACVPR voting privileges.

Fellow
Shall be qualified as a Member for at least two consecutive years; attended a minimum of two Annual Meetings; demonstrated high standards of professional development and a commitment to the goals and long-range activities of the Association; submitted evidence of outstanding performance in some aspect of cardiovascular or pulmonary rehabilitation over a period of at least five years relative to (a) clinical practice, (b) research, and/or (c) professional education in cardiovascular and pulmonary rehabilitation; received recommendations in writing by two Fellows of the Association; and received the approval of the Credentials Committee and the Board of Directors. Fellows have AACVPR voting privileges.

Student Member
Shall be any interested college student currently carrying the equivalent of at least one half of an academic load for one year, as defined by the university or college the person is attending, and one who is studying in a medical or allied health curriculum.

Associate Member
Shall be any person with an interest in cardiovascular and/or pulmonary rehabilitation, but not currently eligible for classification as a Member or Student Member. Dues are established by the Board of Directors and may be changed at its discretion. Associate Member privileges include a subscription to any AACVPR newsletter that may be published and placement on the Association mailing list.